WORKBOOK TO ACCOMPANY

Health Information Technology and Management

RICHARD GARTEE
KIRSTIE DEBIASE
MATT LARDIE
VALERIE LYNN

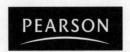

PEARSON

Boston   Columbus   Indianapolis   New York   San Francisco   Upper Saddle River   Amsterdam
Cape Town   Dubai   London   Madrid   Milan   Munich   Paris   Montreal   Toronto   Delhi
Mexico City   Sao Paulo   Sydney   Hong Kong   Seoul   Singapore   Taipei   Tokyo

10 9 8 7 6 5 4

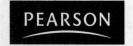

www.pearsonhighered.com

ISBN-13: 978-0-13-212610-6
ISBN-10:   0-13-212610-9

Contents

Introduction

This *Workbook* is designed for use with the textbook *Health Information Technology and Management* by Richard Gartee. Each of the 12 workbook chapters contains activities that correspond to the learning outcomes contained in the textbook. Activities may be assigned as part of regular class work or completed as independent study, depending on the needs of a particular course.

Each *Workbook* chapter includes:

- Learning Outcomes from the textbook with references to related activities within the workbook manual.
- An Introduction that summarizes the main themes from the textbook chapter.
- A variety of activities that test knowledge retention, promote critical thinking, or inspire research and investigation.

Also included in the *Workbook*:

- An Appendix of 10 mock patient records that students will use to complete several of the activities appears at the end of the workbook. Electronic copies of these 10 records, plus an additional 20 mock patient records, may be found on the Companion Website at *www.myhealthprofessionskit.com*.

Note to Instructors—

- Answers to all of the Workbook Activities may be found on the Companion Website at *www.myhealthprofessionskit.com*.

CHAPTER 1
Healthcare Delivery Fundamentals

After completing Chapter 1 from the textbook, you should be able to:	Related Activity in the Workbook
Differentiate ambulatory and acute care facilities	Activity 1-1: Delivery System Matching
Read an organizational chart	Activity 1-2: Create an Organizational Chart
Explain the difference between rehabilitation and long-term facilities	Activity 1-3: Case Studies
Compare the workflows in an inpatient versus outpatient setting	Activity 1-4: Create an Inpatient/Outpatient Venn Diagram
Understand the roles of various direct care providers	Activity 1-5: Who Am I?
Identify the various organizations associated with the healthcare professions	Activity 1-6: Research

INTRODUCTION

Healthcare is provided in a variety of locations and facilities. The biggest differences in facilities are seen between inpatient and outpatient facilities. An outpatient facility provides care to the patient who does not require an overnight stay, whereas an inpatient facility cares for patients who have an illness or injury that is severe enough to require them to stay overnight for one or more days.

Healthcare professions can be broadly categorized into two groups: (1) direct care providers, who provide healthcare services directly to the patient, and (2) nonclinical allied health professionals, who serve the healthcare system but do not provide patient care. To best understand the work flow in any work setting whether inpatient or outpatient, an organizational chart is used to illustrate the managerial relationship between the various jobs shown in the boxes on the chart. In an organizational chart the most responsible position is listed at the top, the next level of management below that person, then the next and so forth.

ACTIVITY 1-1: DELIVERY SYSTEM MATCHING

Name: _____

Date: _____

Course: _____

Learning Outcome

Differentiate ambulatory and acute care facilities.

Directions

For each diagnosis, procedure, or location listed below, indicate whether it is affiliated with either an outpatient (ambulatory care) facility (OP) or an inpatient (acute care) facility (IP), or both (IP/OP). Use a medical dictionary or online resource for help identifying medical terminology, if necessary. Explain your answer for each by providing a rationale.

1. Occupational therapist _____

   Rationale:

   _____

   _____

   _____

2. Bariatric surgery _____

   Rationale:

   _____

   _____

   _____

3. Dentist _____

   Rationale:

   _____

   _____

   _____

4. Mammogram _____

   Rationale:

   _____

   _____

   _____

5. Emergency department _____

   Rationale:

   _____

   _____

   _____

6. Deep vein thrombosis _____
   Rationale:
   _____
   _____
   _____

7. Public health nurse _____
   Rationale:
   _____
   _____
   _____

8. MRI or CAT scan _____
   Rationale:
   _____
   _____
   _____

9. Speech therapist _____
   Rationale:
   _____
   _____
   _____

10. Labor and delivery _____
    Rationale:
    _____
    _____
    _____

11. Pneumonia _____
    Rationale:
    _____
    _____
    _____

12. Lab _____
    Rationale:
    _____
    _____
    _____

13. Chiropractor _____
    Rationale:
    _____
    _____
    _____

14. Radiation therapy _____
    Rationale:
    _____
    _____
    _____

15. Dehydration _____
    Rationale:
    _____
    _____
    _____

16. Physical therapy _____
    Rationale:
    _____
    _____
    _____

17. Diabetic foot ulcer _____
    Rationale:
    _____
    _____
    _____

18. Renal dialysis _____
    Rationale:
    _____
    _____
    _____

19. Internal fixation of a fracture _____
    Rationale:
    _____
    _____
    _____

20. Physicians _____
    Rationale:
    _____
    _____
    _____

ACTIVITY 1-2: CREATE AN ORGANIZATIONAL CHART

Name: _____

Date: _____

Course: _____

Learning Outcome

Read an organizational chart.

Directions

Create an organizational chart using Microsoft Word (choose Insert, then Diagram) or download a free organizational chart from www.SmartDraw.com and select the *Basic Org Chart* model. Once you have downloaded your chart, insert the following job titles of the Health Information Management department where they belong.

Health records clerk

Transcriptionist

HIPAA compliance officer

Office manager

Utilization review coordinator

Health information management (HIM) director

Coding and billing specialist

Facilities manager

ACTIVITY 1-3: CASE STUDIES

Name: _____

Date: _____

Course: _____

Learning Outcome

Explain the difference between rehabilitation and long-term facilities.

Directions

Read the following case studies and decide whether the patient should be transferred to a *long-term care facility* or to a *rehabilitation facility*. Use a medical dictionary or online reference if necessary to assist you with unfamiliar medical terminology.

1. The patient is an 89-year-old male with a history of coronary artery disease and hypertension who sustained good health status and was living independently at home until he began exhibiting signs of dementia and profound weakness. He was taken to an acute care hospital in a dehydrated state with a low-grade fever. After study, the patient was found to have a nondisplaced hip fracture and was taken to surgery for open reduction, internal fixation of the hip fracture. During the postoperative hours, he suffered a cerebrovascular accident (CVA). His course continued to worsen, and he developed atrial fibrillation and deep venous thrombosis. He was evaluated and subsequently transferred to a _____.

2. The patient is a 23-year-old female with a three-year addiction to methamphetamines. Her condition has recently worsened, symptomatic with severe weight loss, rapid heartbeats, and hallucinations. Her family has staged an intervention to get her help to hopefully encourage her to enter a

   _____.

3. The patient is a 73-year-old woman whose mental state has been declining rapidly during the past year. At first, the problem was simple forgetfulness about leaving the stove on or washing the laundry incorrectly, but then progressed to accidentally using cleaning products while preparing food or walking outside in freezing weather in a bathrobe because of paranoia about men being in the house. Soon, she was unable to remember words and was falling asleep while doing activities, soiling herself, and withdrawing her money from the bank and hiding it all around the house to keep it safe. Her loved ones began to worry about her physical safety, and it soon became obvious that she was not able to shop or prepare food for herself any longer, bathe, or maintain clean clothes and a clean living environment. After much counseling with a trusted healthcare professional the family decided the best decision was to transfer her to a _____.

4. The patient is a 45-year-old woman who has always struggled with being overweight. Her husband recently divorced her for a much younger, thinner woman, which caused the patient to spiral into severe depression. She takes antidepressants and sees her therapist three times a week but has begun starving herself so she can lose weight "once and for all." The weight-loss plan started out relatively healthy, but has declined to the point where she is eating only one-quarter of the daily recommended nutrients for a woman of her stature. Her hair has begun to fall out in patches, her teeth are loose, her skin is pallid, and her bone structure is protruding under her skin. Her sister has gone with her to her doctor because the patient is extremely fatigued and unable to perform her work duties and her boss ordered her to seek help or be terminated. The doctor has prescribed one month's stay at a _____.

ACTIVITY 1-4: CREATE AN INPATIENT/ OUTPATIENT VENN DIAGRAM

Name: _____

Date: _____

Course: _____

Learning Outcome

Compare the workflows in an inpatient versus outpatient setting.

Directions

Put the following phrases inside the circles where they belong identifying the characteristics of an **Inpatient,** an **Outpatient,** or **Both.**

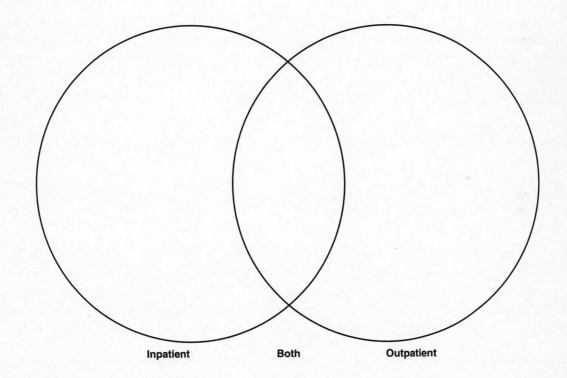

Inpatient   Both   Outpatient

Patient stays overnight

Patient does not stay overnight

Group medical practice

Hospital

Facility measured by number of beds

Facility measured by number of visits or encounters

Comprehensive medical records and medical charts

Current acute care issue on new patient record or chart

Patient "checks in"

Patient registration on first visit

Formal patient admission and discharge process

"New" patient is a status

"Established" patient is a status

Patient has copay

Patient schedules a follow-up appointment

Doctor orders tests, medications, and procedures

ACTIVITY 1-5: WHO AM I?

Name: _____

Date: _____

Course: _____

Learning Outcome

Understand the roles of various direct care providers.

Directions

Read the following descriptions given by direct care providers describing their certifications and job duties, then write their position's title on the line.

1. I am a licensed professional with training in patient care. I graduated from a vocational school and learned how to provide routine care for patients.

   _____

2. I have training and qualifications in pregnancy, childbirth, and postpartum care.

   _____

3. I work collaboratively with a PCP and provide a level of services similar to the physician, including diagnosing the patient and writing prescriptions.

   _____

4. I am the responsible entity in the healthcare continuum with a legal and ethical responsibility for the treatments I provide and those treatments provided by other caregivers under my orders.

   _____

5. I am certified to administer anesthesiology during surgery under the supervision of the medical doctor.

   _____

6. I could take additional tests after licensing to become board certified in my chosen field to add to my credentials and provide other advantages to my profession.

   _____

7. I am licensed to administer medications, perform various medical procedures, and render care to the patient.

   _____

8. I work under the supervision of a physician to ease the physician's workload. I conduct physical exams, diagnose, treat illnesses, order and interpret tests, counsel on preventive healthcare, assist in surgery and write prescriptions.

   _____

ACTIVITY 1-6: RESEARCH

Name: _____

Date: _____

Course: _____

Learning Outcome

Identify the various organizations associated with the healthcare professions.

Directions

Using your preferred search engine (*www.google.com*, *www.bing.com*, *www.yahoo.com*, *www.ask.com*), research up to five organizations that serve healthcare professionals. List their membership benefits, dates of inception, fees, and mission statements. Consider whether membership in each organization may have benefits to you as a student and as a future health information professional.

1. Organization name: _____
   Membership benefits: _____
   Dates of inception: _____
   Fees: _____
   Mission statement: _____
   Benefits: _____

2. Organization name: _____
   Membership benefits: _____
   Dates of inception: _____
   Fees: _____
   Mission statement: _____
   Benefits: _____

3. Organization name: _____
   Membership benefits: _____
   Dates of inception: _____
   Fees: _____
   Mission statement: _____
   Benefits: _____

4. Organization name: _____
   Membership benefits: _____
   Dates of inception: _____
   Fees: _____

Mission statement: _____

Benefits: _____

5. Organization name: _____

   Membership benefits: _____

   Dates of inception: _____

   Fees: _____

   Mission statement: _____

   Benefits: _____

WEBSITE RESOURCES

American Health Information Management Association

www.ahima.org

The American Health Information Management Association (AHIMA) is a nationally recognized organization that is considered to be the leader in health information management (HIM). HIM professionals can join to improve the quality of health records, educate others, advocate for health policies, and network for career advancement. AHIMA also provides certifications in coding, health information management, healthcare privacy and security, and health data analytics.

Allied Health Group

www.alliedhealth.com

Allied Health Group (AHG) was founded to provide staffing for nurse practitioners and physician assistants. Many midlevel providers work with AHG to find employment in quality healthcare opportunities. AHG is Joint Commission certified and the website has many important health links and an online job search engine.

American Hospital Association

www.aha.org

The American Hospital Association (AHA) is a national organization that serves 5,000 hospitals, healthcare systems, networks, and providers as advocates, representatives, and educators on issues, laws, and healthcare research and trends.

U.S. Department of Health and Human Services

www.hhs.gov/about/orgchart

This website shows the organizational chart of the U.S. Department of Health and Human Services. Each title is hyperlinked so the user can read the mission of each position. Users can also learn about career opportunities. Links to the Operating Division home pages are also available at the bottom of the web page.

Journal of the American Medical Association

http://jama.ama-assn.org

The *Journal of the American Medical Association* (JAMA) has been published since 1883 and is an international, peer-reviewed journal published 48 times per year. It is renowned as the most widely circulated medical journal worldwide. The key objective of the JAMA is to promote the science and art of medicine and the betterment of the public's health.

FORE Library

http://library.ahima.org/xpedio/groups/public/documents/web_assets/bok_home.hcsp

The FORE Library is anchored by the AHIMA organization and hosts links to public materials needed by successful professionals in health information management. Items that can be accessed include AHIMA journals, practice briefs, professional tools, HIPAA information, education, records management, patient advocacy and coding information, legislation, and guidelines.

CHAPTER 2
Health Information Professionals

After completing Chapter 2 from the textbook, you should be able to:	Related Activity in the Workbook
Describe the history of health information management organizations	Activity 2-1: Timeline
Differentiate the roles of health information professionals	Activity 2-2: Chain Link
Describe the organizational hierarchy of HIM and IT departments	Activity 2-3: What Is a Project Manager?
Compare various nonclinical allied healthcare occupations	Activity 2-4: Quadrant Graphic
Explain the role of a project manager	Activity 2-3: What Is a Project Manager?
Understand how skill sets from multiple disciplines can help you in your career	Activity 2-5: Job Search

INTRODUCTION

Nonclinical allied health professions are those occupations in healthcare that do not involve providing medical or diagnostic services to the patient; instead, people in these professions handle and safeguard the medical information vital to those who do provide direct services. This category includes all HIS, IT, HIM, and HIT professions. Some examples are medical office managers, registration and scheduling clerks, medical record clerks, transcriptionists, computer system analysts, IT managers, and billing and coding specialists. Nonclinical allied health professionals impact the ability of the clinic to care for the patient by their attention to accuracy and detail. These professionals ensure successful operation of the healthcare delivery system.

ACTIVITY 2-1: TIMELINE

Name: _____

Date: _____

Course: _____

Learning Outcome

Describe the history of health information management organizations.

Directions

Write the corresponding letter from the list below in each arrow to reflect the date of each event.

A. American Medical Record Association established

B. Association of Record Librarians of North America established

C. Health Insurance Portability and Accountability Act (HIPAA) established

D. "As is" records

E. American Health Information Management Association (AHIMA) established

F. American College of Surgeons (ACS) initiative

G. AARL name officially established

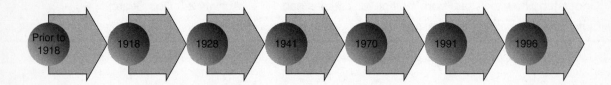

ACTIVITY 2-2: CHAIN LINK

Name: _____

Date: _____

Course: _____

Learning Outcome

Differentiate the roles of health information professionals.

Directions

Health information management (HIM) professionals are linked in a linear chain so they can work together to make the healthcare profession run smoothly. The picture below helps demonstrate the interdependence of the different titles and functions. Using the chain and the words below, list job titles, the acronyms, and the main responsibilities associated with each HIM profession.

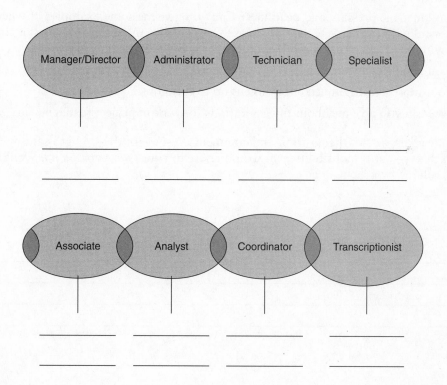

ACTIVITY 2-3: WHAT IS A PROJECT MANAGER?

Name: _____

Date: _____

Course: _____

Learning Outcomes

Describe the organizational hierarchy of HIM and IT departments.

Explain the role of a project manager.

Directions

Find a project manager at a local healthcare facility and interview this person about his or her job. Write two paragraphs explaining the role(s) of a project manager. Some sample questions are provided to get you started:

1. What motivates you? How do you motivate others?
2. How do you manage pressure and deadlines? Can you give me some examples of when you have been successful with the management of stress? Can you give me some examples of struggles you have had with the stress of being a project manager and what you have done to overcome them?
3. How do you handle change?
4. What is your most significant accomplishment up to this point?
5. What advice can you give me about my aspirations to work in project management?

Be sure to include all aspects of the position and comment on some of the strengths and weaknesses associated with this type of responsibility as it would relate to your own personality. Would you be effective in this role? Why or why not?

Notes:

_____

_____

_____

_____

ACTIVITY 2-4: QUADRANT GRAPHIC

Name: _____

Date: _____

Course: _____

Learning Outcome

Compare various nonclinical allied healthcare occupations.

Directions

Chapter 2 explores many nonclinical allied healthcare occupations. Their main functions are broken down into four quadrants. Fill in the corresponding blank quadrants with the job titles and responsibilities as related.

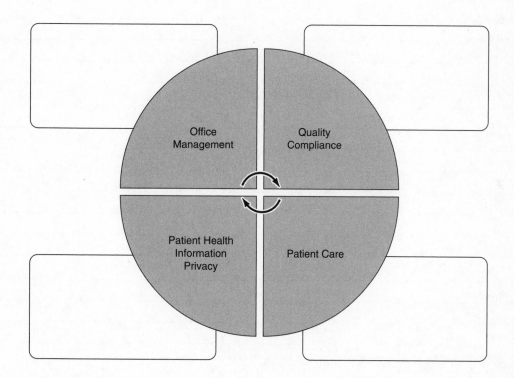

ACTIVITY 2-5: JOB SEARCH

Name: _____

Date: _____

Course: _____

Learning Outcome

Understand how skill sets from multiple disciplines can help you in your career.

Directions

Perform research online to locate job positions at the local hospitals in your region, or research job positions at the website resources listed at the end of this chapter. Make a list of the reoccurring skill sets employers desire for employees and identify how cross training among multiple disciplines can open up the doors for more opportunity in your future career.

Job Title: _____

Skills Required: _____

_____

_____

Job Title: _____

Skills Required: _____

_____

_____

Job Title: _____

Skills Required: _____

_____

_____

Job Title: _____

Skills Required: _____

_____

_____

Common skills among job positions include:

_____

_____

_____

_____

_____

WEBSITE RESOURCES

Association for Healthcare Documentation Integrity

www.ahdionline.org/scriptcontent/index.cfm

The Association for Healthcare Documentation Integrity (AHDI) is the world's largest resource for the latest information on health data capture and documentation. The AHDI sets the standards for education and practice in the field of medical transcription and editing. Transcription professionals can become members, get credentialed, and network within their field to develop professionally and seek additional employment, advice, or tips related to their careers.

National Committee for Quality Assurance

www.ncqa.org

The National Committee for Quality Assurance (NCQA) is a private, not-for-profit organization committed to the continuous improvement in quality healthcare deliverance. On this website information about many programs, publications, events, products, and health education is available. Furthermore, report cards are available on healthcare organizations, plans, and providers. The ratings assigned by the report cards can be selected to obtain further information regarding an organization's good or poor performance.

Centers for Medicare and Medicaid Services

www.cms.gov

The Centers for Medicare and Medicaid Services (CMS) is the main federal government agency responsible for healthcare. It was formerly known as the Healthcare Financing Agency, an agency of the U.S. Department of Health and Human Services. The CMS administers the federal Medicare and Medicaid programs and is not only the main point of reference for the government coverage programs but also private-sector payers because of their strict yet effective management and reimbursement regulations.

Utilization Review Accreditation Commission

www.urac.org

The Utilization Review Accreditation Commission (URAC) is an independent, nonprofit accreditor founded in 1990 that administers accreditation and certification programs. The URAC started out by developing a common set of quality standards for utilization reviews but has expanded to accredit healthcare plans, programs, websites, and networks within the United States. The URAC website is a valuable resource with links explaining the history of URAC, potential employers, testimonies, education, policy makers, and healthcare organizations.

CHAPTER 3
Accreditation, Regulation, and HIPAA

After completing Chapter 3 from the textbook, you should be able to:	Related Activity in the Workbook
Discuss the importance of accreditation	Activity 3-1: Promo!
Understand HIPAA privacy and security concepts	Activity 3-2: Privacy or Security? Activity 3-6: Release of Information
Apply HIPAA privacy policy in a medical office	Activity 3-3: What If?
Discuss HIPAA security requirements and safeguards	Activity 3-4: Guard Dog
Follow security policy guidelines in a medical facility	Activity 3-5: On-the-Job Training

INTRODUCTION

Healthcare facilities and practitioners are licensed and regulated by federal, state, and local governments and laws. Government regulation influences healthcare delivery first by requiring licensure of both the facilities and their providers, and secondly by requiring them to meet certain conditions to participate in programs such as Medicare that reimburse them for treating patients. Participating providers and facilities are subject to inspection and audit by CMS as well as other insurance programs. Compliance with standards set by the Joint Commission, CAP, CARF, and other approved organizations can earn the facilities a *deemed status*, meaning the accredited facility is deemed to have complied with CMS Conditions of Participation (COP). The Health Insurance Portability and Accountability Act or HIPAA was passed in 1996 and has four distinct components: transactions and code sets, uniform identifiers, privacy, and security. HIPAA regulates health plans, clearinghouses, and healthcare providers as "covered entities" in regard to these four areas.

ACTIVITY 3-1: PROMO!

Name: _____

Date: _____

Course: _____

Learning Outcome

Discuss the importance of accreditation.

Directions

Becoming accredited by the Joint Commission is a voluntary option for healthcare insurance plans and agencies, but many find compliance with the commission's standards beneficial. Review the benefits of accreditation discussed in Chapter 3 and visit the Joint Commission website at *www.jointcommission.org/*. Then design an advertisement, poster, PowerPoint presentation, or radio/TV info-commercial that outlines the benefits of Joint Commission accreditation and certification. Make it exciting and appealing to the listener or reader and be sure to include as many components as possible of the benefits that accreditation can provide.

Benefits of accreditation include:

_____

_____

_____

_____

_____

_____

_____

_____

_____

_____

_____

_____

ACTIVITY 3-2: PRIVACY OR SECURITY?

Name: _____

Date: _____

Course: _____

Learning Outcome

Understand HIPAA privacy and security concepts.

Directions

For each of the following statements, put *P* for *privacy* or *S* for *security* or *B* for *both* to better understand how the two concepts are complementary and unique.

1. This rule covers PHI in electronic communications. _____

2. This rule applies to PHI in electronic, oral, and written form. _____

3. This rule contains provisions that currently require covered entities to adopt certain safeguards for PHI. _____

4. The Office of Civil Rights (OCR) enforces this rule. _____

5. The CMS enforces this rule. _____

6. Implementation specifications in this rule are "Required" or "Addressable." _____

7. The largest category of this rule is Administrative Safeguards. _____

8. This rule allows covered providers and health plans to disclose protected health information to business associates if the providers or plans obtain written assurances that it will only be used for the purposes for which it was engaged by the covered entity. _____

9. This rule grants healthcare professionals the discretion to allow or deny a parent access to a minor's PHI based on their professional judgment. _____

10. This rule requires covered entities to treat an individual's personal representative as the individual with respect to uses and disclosures of the individual's protected health information and rights. _____

11. Under this rule the term *consent* is only concerned with the use of the patient's information and should not be confused with consent for the treatment itself. _____

ACTIVITY 3-3: WHAT IF?

Name: _____

Date: _____

Course: _____

Learning Outcome

Apply HIPAA privacy policy in a medical office.

Directions

Imagine you are a health information management professional in a medical office. Work with a partner or independently to brainstorm responses to the following "what if" scenarios. Make notes and be prepared to share them with the class.

What Would You Do If...?

1. Someone you knew came into your medical office for treatment. How would you greet the person? Would you initiate conversation? What if you saw the person later outside of the medical office?

   _____

   _____

   _____

   _____

   _____

2. A concerned and upset parent called your office wanting to know if her 15-year-old daughter was pregnant.

   _____

   _____

   _____

   _____

   _____

3. You witnessed a coworker taking home a flash drive or laptop with patient private health information on it.

   _____

   _____

   _____

   _____

4. Your computer screen is visible to patients at the front desk window.

   _____

   _____

   _____

_____

_____

5. A nonpatient (pharmaceutical representative, job candidate, etc.) was in the back office area surrounded by PHI and you needed to leave the person alone to go attend to a situation in another room?

_____

_____

_____

_____

6. A paralegal from a law firm is researching a worker's compensation claim and calls asking you to fax all of a patient's medical records to the firm.

_____

_____

_____

_____

ACTIVITY 3-4: GUARD DOG

Learning Outcome

Discuss HIPAA security requirements and safeguards.

Directions

Working independently or in a small group, use the following graphic organizer to define each of the HIPAA safeguards and list characteristics associated with HIPAA compliance in a medical office. Be prepared to present your findings to the class.

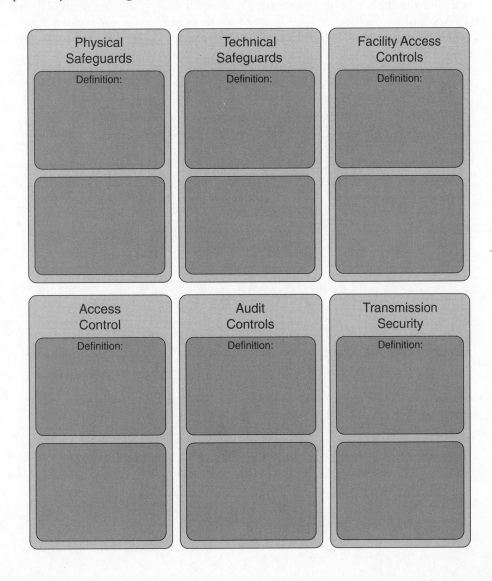

Physical Safeguards — Definition:

Technical Safeguards — Definition:

Facility Access Controls — Definition:

Access Control — Definition:

Audit Controls — Definition:

Transmission Security — Definition:

ACTIVITY 3-5: ON-THE-JOB TRAINING

Name: _____

Date: _____

Course: _____

Learning Outcome

Follow security policy guidelines in a medical facility.

Directions

How would you organize the most important security policy guidelines that all personnel must follow in your medical facility? You have been asked by your supervisor to create a security policy matrix for your facility. Use Figure 3-6 from the textbook as an example when creating your own matrix. Be sure to include the standard, implementation specifications, and consequences as outlined in the security standards rules. They can be accessed by visiting the CMS website at *http://www.cms.gov* and then searching for "privacy and security standards."

Notes:

_____

_____

_____

_____

Name: _____

Date: _____

Course: _____

Learning Outcome

Understand HIPAA privacy and security concepts.

Directions

You are a release of information clerk at your local hospital. You receive a fax from another facility requesting that a record to be sent to the patient. Compare this request to the requirements for a request to be HIPAA compliant and decide if you would proceed with the request.

Friendly Health Clinic
1111 E Sunshine Way, Anywhere, ID 83776
(208) 378-5566

Patient Name:	Robertson, Amy	DOB:	11/7/xx
SSN:	519-53-4478	Phone Number:	208 431-3259

Information Requested: The patient has requested she be sent copies of her entire record.

Send to: Amy Robertson
1604 E Parent Loop
Valley View, ID 83752

This authorization expires 90 days from the date of the signature below. I may revoke this authorization in writing at any time by sending written notification to the Director of HIM. I understand that once the above information is disclosed, it may be redisclosed by the recipient and the information may not be protected by federal privacy laws or regulations.

Amy Robertson   _____   2/9/2010
Patient Signature   Date

Fax transmission received by the HIM department 10/2/2010 at 1130 a.m.

---

1. If you do proceed, what steps are required to fulfill this request?

   _____

   _____

   _____

2. If you do not proceed, what will you do? Discuss.

   _____

   _____

   _____

WEBSITE RESOURCES

Joint Commission

www.jointcommission.org

The Joint Commission monitors more than 16,000 healthcare organizations and programs in the United States. It is also an accreditation and certification agency committed to a high standard of quality, safety, and performance improvement. This website has numerous links to career opportunities, accreditation and certification programs, publications, events, and reports.

National Institutes of Health ListServ

https://list.nih.gov

This website is used to read, post, or manage notifications regarding the latest updates and changes to the HIPAA regulations. Interested parties can sign up to receive this information via an e-mail address.

U.S. Department of Health and Human Services

www.hhs.gov/hipaafaq

At this U.S. Department of Health and Human Services website, you can find answers to the most frequently asked questions (FAQs) about HIPAA.

U.S. Food and Drug Administration

www.fda.gov

The U.S. Food and Drug Administration (FDA) is an extension of the U.S. Department of Health and Human Services. It is dedicated to informing the public about health issues and nutrition. The FDA also regulates safety and compliance regarding medical devices, vaccines, tobacco, cosmetics, and radiation-emitting products.

Centers for Disease Control and Prevention

www.cdc.gov

The Centers for Disease Control and Prevention website covers many health and safety topics such as emergency preparedness and response, environmental concerns, and workplace and travelers' health. It also has many publications including the *Morbidity and Mortality Weekly Report* (MMWR), which is helpful for coding ICD-9-CM codes. The website is also available in Spanish.

Commission on Accreditation of Rehabilitation Facilities

www.carf.org

The Commission on Accreditation of Rehabilitation Facilities (CARF) is an independent, nonprofit organization committed to the accreditation of rehabilitation facilities, providers, services, and programs within the healthcare community. The website has links to education, publications, catalogs, newsletters, conferences, and field reviews of standards.

CHAPTER 4
Fundamentals of Information Systems

After completing Chapter 4 from the textbook, you should be able to:	Related Activity in the Workbook
Understand fundamental concepts of computers	Activity 4-1: Virtual Shopping Spree
Discriminate between hardware and software	Activity 4-2: Piracy Ethics
Define computer input and output	Activity 4-3: Crossword Puzzle
Discuss components of a database	Activity 4-4: Morse Code
Compare different types of computer data and explain relational data	Activity 4-5: My Computer
Describe different types of computer networks	Activity 4-6: Acronym Match
Understand how a wireless network functions	Activity 4-7: Diagram
Understand how interoperability standards help disparate systems exchange data	Activity 4-8: Write It Out!

INTRODUCTION

Computer systems are generally discussed in terms of two components: *hardware* and *software*. Hardware refers to the components you can physically see and touch, whereas software refers to the operating system and application programs that provide instructions to the hardware to process the information the computer receives and stores. Multiple computers can be linked together into a *network*. This allows them to communicate with each other and share files and information.

The fundamental unit of modern computing is called a *bit*. Bits are grouped together in logical units, the most common of which is called a *byte*. There are eight bits in one byte. The smallest units of text data are characters which are limited to letters, numbers, a space, and punctuation marks. Computer *data* is information that can be stored and retrieved. Data is stored on disk drives in files and databases. Data is input into the computer using a keyboard, mouse, touch screen, microphone, camera, or scanner or can be directly transferred from another computer or medical device using an electronic data interface. Computer output devices include printers, screens or monitors, and computer output to laser disk.

Computer software consists of program instructions that enable us to work. Operating systems and network software control computer hardware, input/output devices, and communications with other computers. When a facility uses application software from many different vendors for their electronic health records, it is necessary to use a data exchange standard such as HL7 to electronically transfer information between the various applications.

ACTIVITY 4-1: VIRTUAL SHOPPING SPREE

Name: _____

Date: _____

Course: _____

Learning Outcome

Understand fundamental concepts of computers.

Directions

Research various magazine, newspaper, and Internet advertisements for new computers on sale in your area, focusing on Dell, Hewlett-Packard, and Mac. Print or photocopy the advertisements and circle all of the features each computer includes. Next create a chart that delineates the various features you learned about in Chapter 4 of the textbook, such as RAM, operating system and application software, peripheral devices included, and so on. Or use the following sample table.

Comparison Worksheet			
	Dell	**HP**	**Apple**
What is the price of the computer?			
Who manufactured the microprocessor?			
What is the processor model and speed?			
How much RAM is included?			
What is the maximum RAM capacity?			
What is the hard disk drive capacity?			
What is the speed of the optical drive (or CD, Blu-ray, or DVD drive/burner)?			
Is a monitor included?			
What is the size and resolution of the screen?			
What type of graphics card is included?			
How much memory is on the graphics card?			
How many USB ports are included?			
How many drive bays are filled and how many are available?			
What kinds of expansion slots are available?			
What is the overall weight (notebook only)?			
Which version of the operating system is included?			
Is any other software included?			

	Dell	HP	Apple
What is covered by the manufacturer's warranty?			
Is an extended warranty available?			
Where can I get technical support?			

Now that you have completed your research, describe which computer you would consider purchasing and why. How would this particular computer assist you as a student? How would this particular computer assist you as an HIM professional?

_____

_____

_____

_____

_____

_____

_____

_____

ACTIVITY 4-2: PIRACY ETHICS

Name: _____

Date: _____

Course: _____

Learning Outcome

Discriminate between hardware and software.

Directions

Research the software piracy FAQs at *www.ed.uiuc.edu/wp/copyright-2002/softwarepiracyfaqs.html*. What determines "piracy" can be an ethical dilemma for the public to understand because it does not feel like stealing because what is being stolen is intangible, unlike physical computer hardware.

1. What is the definition of software piracy?

   _____

   _____

   _____

   _____

2. What exactly does the law say about copying software?

   _____

   _____

   _____

   _____

3. Can I take a piece of software owned by my school and install it on my personal computer at home?

   _____

   _____

   _____

   _____

4. Can I purchase a single, licensed copy of a piece of software and load it onto several machines?

   _____

   _____

   _____

   _____

5. What are the maximum civil penalties for copyright infringement?

   _____

   _____

   _____

   _____

6. What are the maximum criminal penalties for copyright infringement?

_____

_____

_____

_____

7. What are my responsibilities as a consumer?

_____

_____

_____

_____

8. Design a public service announcement to educate the public about the illegality of software piracy, the ramifications, the civil penalties, and prevention tactics.

ACTIVITY 4-3: CROSSWORD PUZZLE

Name: _____

Date: _____

Course: _____

Learning Outcome

Define computer input and output.

Directions

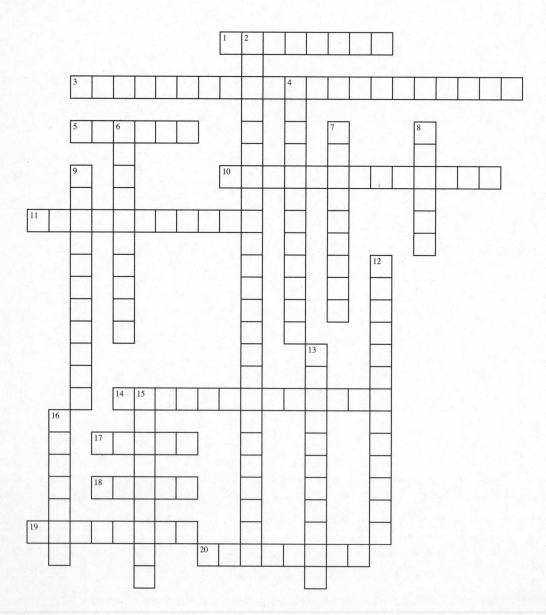

Across

1. This peripheral device processes output and makes it audible.
3. The brain of the computer.
5. This input device enters images into the computer.
10. This device can be internally or externally mounted on the system unit and is the primary storage device.
11. This card is used to connect a computer to a network or cable Internet connection.
14. This device plugs directly into a USB port on the computer system unit to read or store data.
17. This device is designed to manipulate on-screen graphics and controls.
18. This establishes an Internet connection and may be either internal or external.
19. This input device enters text and numbers into the computer.
20. This computer is compact and lightweight with its keyboard, monitor, and system in one unit.

Down

2. Typically used as an electronic appointment book, address book, calculator, notepad, or phone.
6. This peripheral device interprets and inserts voice data into the computer.
7. A large and expensive computer capable of simultaneously processing data for hundreds or thousands of users.
8. This device serves the computers on a network by supplying them with data.
9. Contains the processor.
12. Used to store data on a computer or to share data among computers and is both an input and an output device.
13. Powerful desktop computer designed for specialized tasks.
15. Sends sound signals to internal speakers.
16. An output device that produces computer-generated text or graphics on paper.

ACTIVITY 4-4: MORSE CODE

Name: _____

Date: _____

Course: _____

Learning Outcome

Discuss components of a database.

Directions

Part 1

The task of understanding the components of a database is similar to learning to speak a different language. How skilled are you at decoding? Are you as quick and efficient as a computer? Go to the website *www.learnmorsecode.com* and use the International Morse Code to write your full name, date of birth, and school name. Now go to the website *www.asciitable.com* and write your full name, date of birth, and school name. Share your findings and the experience of decoding with your classmates.

Part 2

Using the following patient names, birth dates, primary care physician names, and insurance carriers, organize the data in Excel. Use Figure 4-8 from the textbook as an example.

1. Alejandra Torres
   #444756289A
   Medicaid
   April 22, 1979
   Dr. Jay Wani

2. Chad Stevens
   #XLJH4897555
   Blue Shield of California
   March 15, 1963
   Dr. Jeannine Urquico

3. Cristophe Legrandejacques
   #56987
   PacificCare
   February 27, 1947
   Dr. Kevin Bowers

4. Wendy Young
   #9562789156YUL
   HealthNet
   May 5, 1999
   Dr. Charles Montoya

5. Howard Spoeneman
   #89874124764A
   Medicare
   September 27, 1922
   Dr. William Purnell

ACTIVITY 4-5: MY COMPUTER

Name: _____

Date: _____

Course: _____

Learning Outcome

Compare different types of computer data and explain relational data.

Directions

Start up your computer (either at home, work, or school) and open the Start menu. List at least 10 programs you have, what data they use, and their functions.

Program Name	Data Used	Function

Were any programs unfamiliar to you?

_____

_____

_____

How might you learn about the different functions of unfamiliar programs?

_____

_____

_____

Open up the My Documents or My Pictures folders and write down at least six file name extensions you have used. Share your findings with your class and note any commonalities or differences.

1. _____

2. _____

3. _____

4. _____

5. _____

6. _____

ACTIVITY 4-6: ACRONYM MATCH

Name: _____

Date: _____

Course: _____

Learning Outcome

Describe different types of computer networks.

Directions

Part 1

Match the following computer network names with the appropriate definition from the lettered list.

1. LAN _____
2. WAN _____
3. Internet _____
4. SSL or VPN _____
5. Wireless _____

A. These networks cover large geographic areas using telecommunication lines to connect into one large private network. It uses two types of lines: leased lines and frame relay.

B. Computers connected by a network serving just the organization or facility in which they are located. This network can be managed locally and is designed to keep data very secure.

C. This network is connected through a radio transceiver called an access point, which is actually wired to the router like other network nodes.

D. This secures and protects information by encrypting the transmission and then decrypting the receipt of the message.

E. This is a worldwide public network, which can be accessed by any computer anywhere and is a network of networks.

Part 2

What types of networks are used at the following familiar places?

1. Starbucks _____
2. Airport _____
3. Medical office _____
4. School _____
5. Insurance company _____
6. Bank _____
7. Library _____
8. Supermarket _____
9. Retail store _____
10. Department of motor vehicles _____

ACTIVITY 4-7: DIAGRAM

Name: _____

Date: _____

Course: _____

Learning Outcome

Understand how a wireless network functions.

Directions

Label each picture by filling in the blanks.

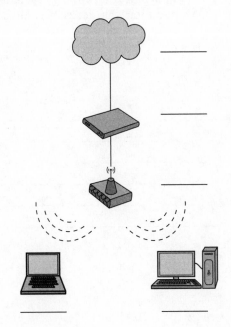

ACTIVITY 4-8: WRITE IT OUT!

Name: _____

Date: _____

Course: _____

Learning Outcome

Understand how interoperability standards help disparate systems exchange data.

Directions

Write a short essay (1 to 1½ pages) on how interoperability standards help different systems exchange data. Be sure to include the two concepts important to healthcare systems, define data elements and data sets and their functions, HL7 and CCOW, and their characteristics and also describe how interoperability is maintained.

Notes:

_____

_____

_____

_____

_____

_____

WEBSITE RESOURCES

Albion.com

www.albion.com/netiquette

This website discusses at length the manners and rules associated with online communication.

National Committee on Vital and Health Statistics

http://ncvhs.hhs.gov/

The National Committee on Vital and Health Statistics has public meetings and serves as an advisory board to the Secretary of the Health and Human Services department. The committee makes recommendations and researches all areas associated with healthcare and reform. It shows how data collection using technology impacts healthcare in many different ways.

National Cancer Data Base

www.facs.org/cancer/ncdb/index.html

The National Cancer Data Base (NCDB) is a joint program of the Commission on Cancer and the American Cancer Society. The NCDB compiles all research and results on approved cancer programs in the United States. It also hosts a tracking system on all cancer data officially collected and reported to the national registry.

Health Level Seven

www.hl7.org

The Health Level Seven (HL7) website has news about ANSI-approved standards and initiatives and is a not-for-profit volunteer organization. Members may join and become committee members responsible for the review and revision of standards.

CHAPTER 5
Healthcare Records

After completing Chapter 5 from the textbook, you should be able to:	Related Activity in the Workbook
Discuss the functions that healthcare records serve	Activity 5-1: Making a List and Checking It Twice
Explain the difference between primary and secondary health records	Activity 5-2: First or Second? Activity 5-8: Abstracting Records
Identify different forms used to record patient information	Activity 5-3: Form Control Activity 5-8: Abstracting Records Activity 5-9: Master Patient Index
Discuss standard data elements and standard data sets	Activity 5-4: Data Relationship
Explain how health records assist in the continuity of care	Activity 5-5: Talk It Out!
Define a RHIO	Activity 5-6: Online Research
Describe the various forms of telemedicine	Activity 5-7: The Shapes of Telemedicine
Explain an E-visit	Activity 5–7: The Shapes of Telemedicine

INTRODUCTION

Healthcare records have many purposes, the most important of which is the patient's care. Data and information are not the same thing. Data are records of facts. Information is data in a useful form that conveys meaning. Patient health record data consists of *administrative and demographic* data and *clinical* data. Administrative data includes a number of legal documents signed by patients or their representative. Demographic data is often gathered on paper forms, and then transferred into the computer by the registration clerk. Clinical data include documents created by the patient, nurses, clinicians, and other providers.

HIM professionals seek to ensure uniform quality patient records. Some of the ways to accomplish this are to use standardized data elements, data sets, and HIM policies and procedures. Patients are also creating personal health records through neutral online entities that allow them to make their records available to different providers they visit. Telemedicine uses communication technology to deliver medical care to a patient in another location and can provide high-level medical expertise to remote and rural areas. E-visits are conducted over the Internet and are being used in some states to allow the patient to be treated by a clinician for nonurgent health problems without having to go to the clinician's office.

ACTIVITY 5-1: MAKING A LIST
AND CHECKING IT TWICE

Name: _____

Date: _____

Course: _____

Learning Outcome

Discuss the functions that healthcare records serve.

Directions

Make a list describing all of the functions that healthcare records serve. Be sure to include both primary and secondary records.

_____

_____

_____

_____

_____

_____

_____

_____

_____

_____

_____

_____

ACTIVITY 5-2: FIRST OR SECOND?

Name: _____

Date: _____

Course: _____

Learning Outcome

Explain the difference between primary and secondary health records.

Directions

Read the following questions and identify whether this type of information would be found in a primary (P) medical record, a secondary (S) medical record, or both (B).

1. This record has information gathered directly from the patient by the provider. _____

2. This record is used in billing. _____

3. This record is used in research. _____

4. This record is used for patient care. _____

5. This record is used for quality improvement. _____

6. This record is a legal document. _____

7. This record is used for abstracting purposes. _____

8. This record contains information from diagnostic tests or medical devices. _____

ACTIVITY 5-3: FORM CONTROL

Name: _____

Date: _____

Course: _____

Learning Outcome

Identify different forms used to record patient information.

Directions

Go to the appendix of 10 patient records that is located at the end of this workbook. Locate an example of each of the following forms and write that patient's name on the line as indicated.

1. **Face sheet**

   Patient Name: _____

2. **SOAP notes**

   Patient Name: _____

3. **Pathology report**

   Patient Name: _____

4. **Physician's orders and progress notes**

   Patient Name: _____

5. **Nursing flow sheet**

   Patient Name: _____

6. **Physical assessment data**

   Patient Name: _____

7. **Nursing notes**

   Patient Name: _____

8. **Consent form**

   Patient Name: _____

9. **Preoperative checklist**

   Patient Name: _____

10. **Discharge summary**

    Patient Name: _____

11. **Treatment record**

    Patient Name: _____

12. **Discharge instructions**

    Patient Name: _____

ACTIVITY 5-4: DATA RELATIONSHIP

Name: _____

Date: _____

Course: _____

Learning Outcome

Discuss standard data elements and standard data sets.

Directions

Under each label write the definition, characteristics, and examples for all parts of data and its uses in health information management. What does each one require, how are they distinct from each other, and what are the standards?

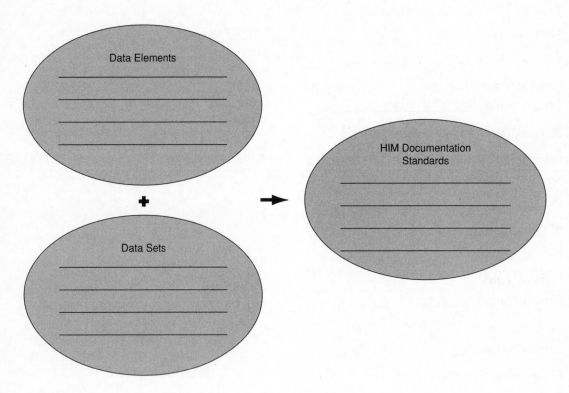

ACTIVITY 5-5: TALK IT OUT!

Name: _____

Date: _____

Course: _____

Learning Outcome

Explain how health records assist in the continuity of care.

Directions

Review the following questions, select one or two, and use them to create a quick, effective 3- to 5-minute debate supporting, explaining, or defending your position to your classmates.

Questions:

1. How do health records assist in the continuity of care?
2. What is the most effective way to facilitate continuity of care among all of the different departments in a health facility serving the same patient?
3. What would you do as the manager of a health information management department to ensure smooth transitions and continuity of care for your patients?
4. What is your personal opinion on RHIOs and the IDN?
5. Describe your own experiences with continuity of care, or lack thereof, during times when you have been a patient.

Notes:

_____

_____

_____

_____

_____

_____

_____

_____

Next, stage a debate with a classmate who has selected the same question as you, but has a different opinion than yours.

ACTIVITY 5-6: ONLINE RESEARCH

Name: _____

Date: _____

Course: _____

Learning Outcome

Define a RHIO.

Directions

Visit the HIMSS website at *http://himss.org*. Search this website to learn more about RHIOs and answer the following questions.

1. What is a RHIO?

   _____

   _____

2. What is an HIE?

   _____

   _____

3. How are RHIOs and HIEs different?

   _____

   _____

4. What are the objectives of RHIOs and HIEs?

   _____

   _____

   _____

   _____

5. What are the benefits of RHIOs?

   _____

   _____

   _____

   _____

6. What challenges do RHIO face?

   _____

   _____

   _____

   _____

   Next create a PowerPoint presentation designed to educate others about this information.

ACTIVITY 5-7: THE SHAPES OF TELEMEDICINE

Name: _____

Date: _____

Course: _____

Learning Outcomes

Describe the various forms of telemedicine.

Explain an E-visit.

Directions

1. Use the following table to list the three main types of telemedicine, and then provide two characteristics of each type.

Telemedicine			
Type	1.	2.	3.
Example			
Example			

2. Visit the websites of telemedicine associations to learn more about telemedicine. What are some issues related to telemedicine that are currently in the news? Write a short research report describing one of the topics that interests you the most. Suggestions for websites include *www.americantelemed.org*, *http://tie.telemed.org*, and *www.nlm.nih.gov*.

3. Perform an Internet search to learn more about E-visits and view some simulations. Then answer the following questions.

   a. How accurate do you think the diagnosis from this type of visit would be?
   b. Would you prefer this type of doctor's visit over a personal one? Why or why not?
   c. How did you feel speaking to this doctor?
   d. Would you recommend this to others? Why or why not?

Share your personal experiences in a class discussion.

Sites to try:

www.justanswer.com

https://www.relayhealth.com

ACTIVITY 5-8: ABSTRACTING RECORDS

Name: _____

Date: _____

Course: _____

Learning Outcomes

Explain the difference between primary and secondary health records.

Identify different forms used to record patient information.

Directions

Abstracting is the collection of data for a particular purpose. Abstracted data is placed in secondary sources of health information, such as the master patient index, physician index, disease index, and procedure index. These indices are used to generate statistics related to the care being provided by the facility and they can be used in business decision-making processes. Another reason to abstract data is to support medical research, contribute to a variety of registries, and maintain compliance with various regulations.

For this activity, you may abstract either ER or OP patient records, or your instructor may decide. Once you determine which record type you will be abstracting, either photocopy and use the forms included in Forms section of the appendix, or if you have access to the Internet, select the appropriate link and print and complete the data abstract for your record. Use the ten mock patient records located in the appendix to complete this activity. Note that you may also use the additional twenty mock patient records that are located on myhealthprofessionskit (see your textbook for registration information) if you would like additional practice.

For ER records, use form NHAMCS-100(ED) located in the Forms section of the appendix, or print the form at the following link: www.cdc.gov/NCHS/data/ahcd/nhamcs100ed_2009.pdf.

Record Number	Service Type
410032	ER
410025	ER
410026	ER

For OP Surgery records, use form NSAS-5 located in the Forms section of the appendix or print the form at the following link: www.cdc.gov/nchs/data/hdasd/nsas_participant/nsas5.pdf.

Record Number	Service Type
410028	OPS
410030	OPS
410024	OPS

ACTIVITY 5-9: MASTER PATIENT INDEX

Name: _____

Date: _____

Course: _____

Learning Outcome

Identify different forms used to record patient information.

Directions

Utilize the mock patient records located in the appendix to abstract the information indicated on the master patient index (MPI) card shown below. This type of card was used by healthcare facilities until computerized registration systems became widely used. Although the majority of facilities no longer maintain a paper card type of system, the information collected remains the same.

Note that you will need to photocopy the form below in order to complete this exercise; another copy appears in the Forms section in the appendix. Note that you may also use the additional twenty mock patient records that are located on myhealthprofessionskit (see your textbook for registration information) if you would like additional practice.

Patient Last Name	Patient First Name	Patient Middle Initial	Record Number	Gender	Race

Address	City	State	Zip	DOB	Age

Mother's Maiden Name	SSN		Place of Birth	

Date & Time of Admission	Date & Time of Discharge	Provider	Service Type	Discharge Status

WEBSITE RESOURCES

Computer-based Patient Record Institute

www.cpri.org

This website is a research hub for the Computer-based Patient Record Institute. It uses the information gathered from numerous patient records to identify trends, network, and inform of changes.

Office of Civil Rights

www.hhs.gov/ocr

This website of the Office of Civil Rights informs the public about their civil, HIPAA, and privacy rights and hosts web links related to patient safety concerns.

College of Healthcare Information Management Executives

www.cio-chime.org

The College of Healthcare Information Management Executives (CHIME) is available to foster professional development among HIM executives and to advocate more effective uses for electronic records management in the healthcare field.

Medical Group Management Association

www.mgma.com

The Medical Group Management Association is a professional organization for medical group managers to join. It serves as a support system and provides certifications, networking, and educational information. Membership is currently at 22,500 members.

Professional Association of Health Care Office Management

www.pahcom.com

The Professional Association of Health Care Office Management (PAHCOM) is a national professional organization that provides certification, conferences, education, social networking, and career opportunities for those in medical practice management.

Organization, Storage, and Management of Health Records

After completing Chapter 6 from the textbook, you should be able to:	Related Activity in the Workbook
Explain the various ways in which paper records are organized and stored	Activity 6-1: File It Away
Differentiate source-oriented, problem-oriented, and integrated records	Activity 6-2: Putting It All Together
Compare different methods of filing numeric charts	Activity 6-3: 1-2-3-FILE!
Describe the workflow of charts in the HIM department	Activity 6-4: Go with the Flow
Calculate the space requirements for filing paper charts	Activity 6-5: Figure It Out
Explain the processes involved in document imaging	Activity 6-6: Image Process Activity 6-7: Exploring a Document Image System Activity 6-8: Importing and Cataloging Images Activity 6-9: Retrieving a Scanned Lab Report
Discuss the HIM responsibilities of the legal health record	Activity 6-10: Essay
Describe the AHIMA code of ethics	Activity 6-11: Code of Ethics Presentation

INTRODUCTION

Chapter 6 discussed how the contents of health records can be organized, various ways they are stored, and the process and ethics of managing them. Several standard schemes exist for organizing a paper chart: source-oriented records, problem-oriented records, integrated records, hybrid health records, and loose sheets. Furthermore, paper charts can be filed in any of several methods: alphabetical or numeric using terminal digit filing, middle digit filing, or straight numeric. Color-coded labels can be used with either alphabetical or numeric methods. Medical record numbers are assigned by several different methods: serial numbering, unit numbering, serial unit numbering, and family numbering.

Medical record circulation and storage is the responsibility of the HIM department. Paper charts are filed and retrieved by a member of the HIM team. Document imaging management systems are computer systems that scan and store images of paper documents. Facilities use document imaging systems to complement EHR systems and to replace or eliminate paper charts.

Legal and ethical management of health records is an important function of the HIM department. Ensuring a complete and accurate legal health record is the responsibility of the HIM professional. HIM professionals are not only responsible for the health record but also for managing the release of the information contained in it. The professional standards by which health information professionals conduct themselves are called *ethics*. Healthcare facilities create policies and procedures to provide guidance in the care and handling of confidential records.

ACTIVITY 6-1: FILE IT AWAY

Name: _____

Date: _____

Course: _____

Learning Outcome

Explain the various ways in which paper records are organized and stored.

Directions

Take the following 40 names and medical record numbers and put each one on an index card in the correct sequence for medical records (Last Name, First Name). Then alphabetize each of the cards and turn them in for review to your instructor. After the instructor has reviewed and returned them, put them in order numerically and turn them in again for review to your instructor.

1. Sister LaRhonda Elliston 123456
2. Paula Richmond 123457
3. Ashford O'Runnels 123458
4. Joyce Ludwig 123459
5. Wilfred Roy Le Stadt 123450
6. LaTonya Ellison 123451
7. Randolph Courier 123452
8. Samuel MacElway 123453
9. Joe Porter 123454
10. Jerome Mighty 123446
11. B.A. O'Rourke 123447
12. Franca Departo 123448
13. Bud Osteen 123449
14. Arstelle Lily Letroy 123440
15. Edwina MacGregor 123441
16. Alicia O'Runnil 123444
17. Jesse Garfield 123430
18. Louise Interson 123431
19. Sophia Ganor 123432
20. Tanya Lester-Schmidt 123433
21. Donald Ray Czak 123435
22. Natalie Kline 123434
23. Thomas English 123436
24. Jo Inzinga 123437
25. William Newton 123438
26. Morton Lester 123439
27. Michael Muldoon 123483
28. Robert Feng 123420
29. Frieda Nester 123421
30. Charles Pandapas 123422
31. Sarah Point 123423
32. Edith Perry 123424
33. Frank Lopez 123425
34. Patricia Levi 123426
35. Vito Incosta 123427
36. Roger Peterson 123428
37. Dora Beth Jefferson 123429
38. Daquisha Quarles, II 123480
39. L.L. Huang 123481
40. Lara Laser 123482

ACTIVITY 6-2: PUTTING IT ALL TOGETHER

Name: _____

Date: _____

Course: _____

Learning Outcome

Differentiate source-oriented, problem-oriented, and integrated records.

Directions

Using the following table, fill in at least two characteristics for each medical record filing system to identify the differences and similarities between source-oriented, problem-oriented, and integrated records.

Integrated Record	1. 2.
Problem-Oriented Record	1. 2.
Source-Oriented Record	1. 2.

ACTIVITY 6-3: 1-2-3-FILE!

Name: _____
Date: _____
Course: _____

Learning Outcome

Compare different methods of filing numeric charts.

Directions

Choose ten of the patients used previously in Activity 6-1 and show how you would file them using the alphanumerical, straight numerical, terminal digit, and middle digit filing systems.

Alphanumeric

1. _____
2. _____
3. _____
4. _____
5. _____
6. _____
7. _____
8. _____
9. _____
10. _____

Straight Numeric

1. _____
2. _____
3. _____
4. _____
5. _____
6. _____
7. _____
8. _____
9. _____
10. _____

Terminal Digit

1. _____
2. _____
3. _____
4. _____
5. _____
6. _____
7. _____
8. _____
9. _____
10. _____

Middle Digit

1. _____
2. _____
3. _____
4. _____
5. _____
6. _____
7. _____
8. _____
9. _____
10. _____

ACTIVITY 6-4: GO WITH THE FLOW

Name: _____

Date: _____

Course: _____

Learning Outcome

Describe the workflow of charts in the HIM department.

Directions

Explain in one paragraph the workflow of charts in the HIM department. Where do they start, how are they pulled, where do they move to within the department, and how are they flagged?

_____

_____

_____

_____

_____

_____

_____

_____

_____

ACTIVITY 6-5: FIGURE IT OUT

Name: _____

Date: _____

Course: _____

Learning Outcome

Calculate the space requirements for filing paper charts.

Directions

Using the formulas and the following example, calculate the space requirements for 75,000, 100,000 and 125,000 patients.

Formula: Shelving holding width $\times$ number of shelves per unit = Per unit inches of holding space

Formula: $\dfrac{\text{Per unit inches of holding space}}{\text{Chart average thickness}}$ = Number of files per unit

Formula: $\dfrac{\text{Number of patients}}{\text{Number of files permitted}}$ = Number of units needed

Example:

Patients	40,000
Chart average thickness	0.5" or ½"
Shelving holdings width	46"
Per unit inches of holding space	368
Number of shelves per shelving unit	8
Number of files per unit	736
Number of units needed	55

Problems:

Patients	_____
Chart average thickness	0.5" or ½"
Shelving holdings width	46"
Per unit inches of holding space	_____
Number of shelves per shelving unit	8
Number of files per unit	_____
Number of units needed	_____

ACTIVITY 6-6: IMAGE PROCESS

Name: _____

Date: _____

Course: _____

Learning Outcome

Explain the processes involved in document imaging.

Directions

Fill in the four steps to the process of imaging documents and the procedures that accompany each step.

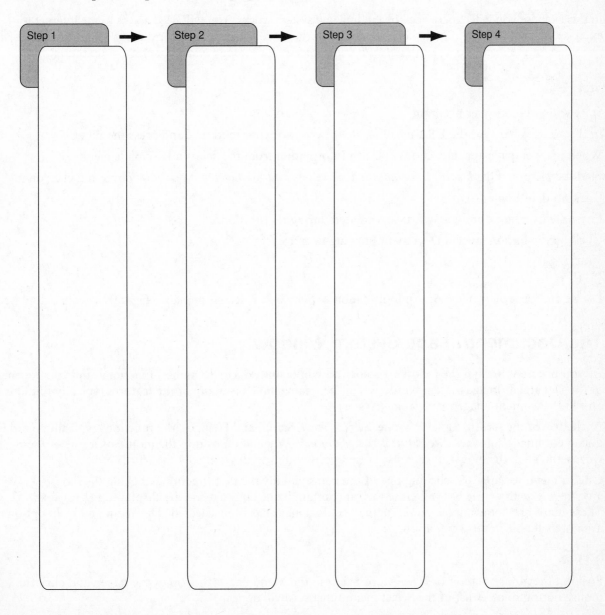

ACTIVITY 6-7: EXPLORING A DOCUMENT IMAGE SYSTEM

Name: _____

Date: _____

Course: _____

Learning Outcome

Explain the processes involved in document imaging.

Directions

In this exercise you will experience how an imaging system works. You will need access to the Internet for this exercise. If you have not already done so, complete the student registration for the MyHealthProfessionsKit provided on the inside cover of the *Health Information Technology and Management* textbook.

Step 1

Start your web browser program.

In the address bar type the URL listed inside the cover of your textbook and press the Enter key.

When the web page appears, choose **Health Information** from the Select a Discipline menu.

Find the picture of the *Health Information Technology and Management* textbook cover and click on it.

Click **Student Login.**

Enter the user name and password you created during registration.

Click on the button labeled **Document Imaging Exercises.**

Step 2

Locate and click on the link **Health Information Activity 6-7.** A screen similar to Figure 6-1 will be displayed.

The Document/Image System Window

As you proceed through the following steps you will be introduced to names, functions, and components of the Document/Image System window. This program simulates many of the features typically found in an EHR document image management system.

At the top of the screen, the words **File, Select, View, Setup,** and **Help** are the functions typically found in document image software. We call this the *Menu bar.* When you position the mouse over one of these words and click the mouse once, a list of functions will drop down below the word.

Once a menu list appears, clicking one of the items will invoke that function. Clicking the mouse anywhere except on the list will close the list. Certain items on the menu are displayed in gray text. These items are not available until a patient or document has been selected. The **Setup** and **Help** options are not available in this simulation.

Step 3

Position the mouse pointer over the word **Select** in the Menu bar at the top of the screen and click the mouse button once. A list of the **Select** menu functions will appear.

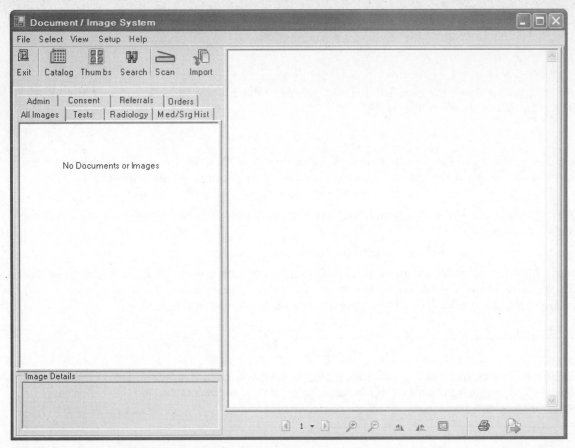

FIGURE 6-1   Document/Image System window.

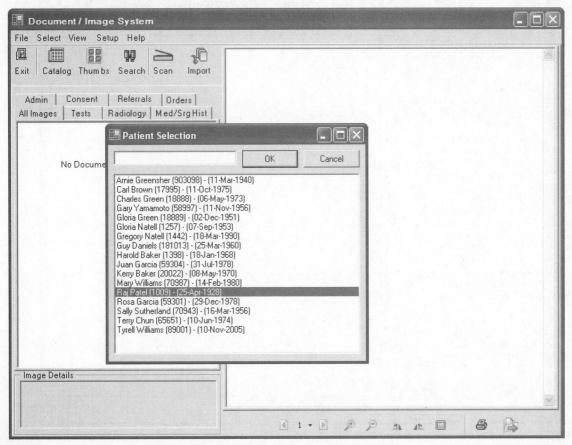

FIGURE 6-2   Selecting Raj Patel from the Patient Selection window.

Step 4

Move the mouse pointer down the list until it is over the word **Patient** and click the mouse to invoke the Patient Selection window shown in Figure 6-2.

Step 5

Locate the patient named Raj Patel in the Patient Selection window. Position the mouse pointer over the patient name and double-click the mouse. (Double-click means to click the mouse button twice, very rapidly.)

Once a patient is selected, the patient's name, age, and sex are displayed in the Title bar at the top of the window (see Figure 6-3).

Compare your screen to Figure 6-3 as you read the following information:

The Toolbar Also located at the top of your screen are a row of icon buttons placed on what is called a *Toolbar*. The purpose of the Toolbar is to allow quick access to commonly used functions. Most Windows programs feature a Toolbar so you may already be familiar with the concept.

Alert

All instructions in these exercises refer to the simulation window. Since you are running this simulation inside a browser, be careful to use the Menu bar and Toolbar inside the simulation window, not the Menu bar or Toolbar of your Internet browser program.

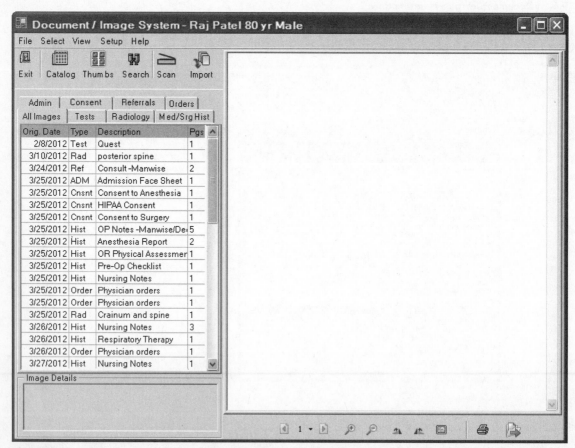

FIGURE 6-3 Title bar at top displays patient's name, age, and sex. The left pane, the Catalog pane, displays a catalog list of documents and images for the selected patient, Raj Patel.

The Catalog Pane The middle portion of the screen is divided into two window panes. The left pane (just below the toolbar) is where a list of cataloged documents is displayed when a patient has been selected. At the top of the Catalog pane there are eight tabs. These look like tabs on file folders. The tabs are used to limit the list to images by category making it easier to find a specific type of image quickly. When the initial tab, "All Images," is active, all available images are listed in date order.

Step 6

Locate the Toolbar in the Document/Image System window. The first icon on the Toolbar is labeled "Exit" and it will close the simulation program and return you to the MyHealthProfessionsKit page. Do not click it yet.

The next two buttons are used to change the display of items in the catalog pane from a list to thumbnails. Thumbnails are small versions of the document or image.

Position your mouse pointer over the **Thumbs** icon on the Toolbar (circled in Figure 6-4) and click your mouse.

Compare your screen to Figure 6-4.

Now position your mouse pointer over the **Catalog** icon on the Toolbar and click your mouse. Your screen should again resemble Figure 6-3.

Step 7

Locate the tab labeled **Med/Srg Hist** above the left pane. Position your mouse pointer over it and click your mouse. The displayed list in the Catalog pane should now be shorter because it is limited to items cataloged in the category of medical/surgical history.

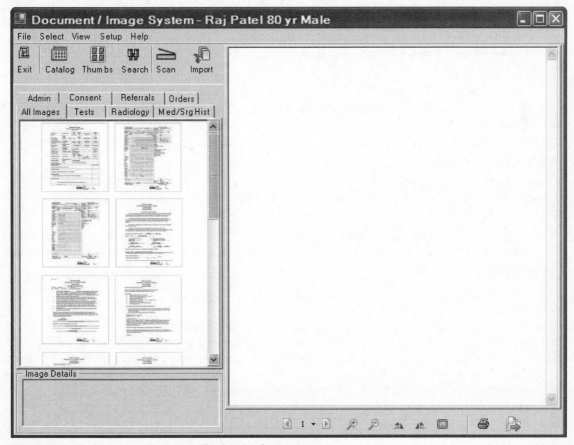

FIGURE 6-4 Catalog pane displaying thumbnails of images.

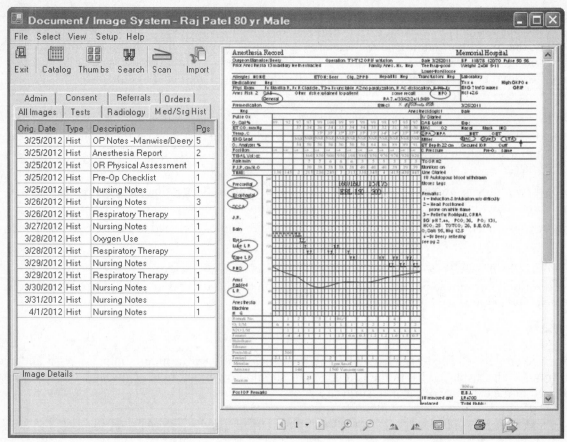

FIGURE 6-5 The Catalog pane shows the catalog for all **Med/Srg Hist** entries, and the right pane, the Image Viewer pane, displays the selected Anesthesia Report.

Step 8

Locate the catalog item **Anesthesia Report** and click on it. Compare your screen to Figure 6-5 as you read the following information.

The Image Viewer Pane   The right pane of the window dynamically displays the corresponding image for a catalog entry that is clicked.

Item Details   Just below the Catalog pane, at the lower left, is a gray panel that displays information about a selected catalog item such as the user who scanned the document, relevant dates, and a longer description of the item.

Image Tools   Just below the Image Viewer pane on the right is a row of icon buttons used to change the displayed image. These changes include the ability to page through multipage documents or to enlarge or reduce the displayed image.

Step 9

Locate the Image Tools buttons just below the Image Viewer pane. The first three icons become active whenever a multipage document is selected. The Anesthesia Report has two pages. Locate and click on the Next Page button (circled in Figure 6-5.) The button displays the next page of a multipage document. The numeral between the two buttons is the page number currently displayed. Your screen should now display the second page of the report and the Image Tool row should display the numeral 2.

The Previous Page button is the first icon in the Image Tools row. Locate it and click on it. The Image Tool row should now display the numeral 1, and the Image Viewer page should again display the first page of the report.

Activity 6-7 is concluded. You may exit and close your browser or proceed to the next activity.

ACTIVITY 6-8: IMPORTING AND CATALOGING IMAGES

Name: _____

Date: _____

Course: _____

Learning Outcome

Explain the processes involved in document imaging.

Directions

The goal of this exercise is to experience how image files are imported and cataloged in a document image system. In this exercise you will catalog a scanned report and a diagnostic image for a patient. You will need access to the Internet for this exercise.

Step 1

If you are still logged in from the previous exercise proceed to Step 2; otherwise, start your web browser program.

In the address bar, type the URL listed inside the cover of your textbook and press the Enter key.

When the web page appears, choose **Health Information** from the Select a Discipline menu.

Find the picture of the *Health Information Technology and Management* textbook cover and click on it.

Click **Student Login.**

Enter the user name and password you created during registration.

Click on the button labeled **Document Imaging Exercises.**

Step 2

Locate and click on the link **Health Information Activity 6-8.** A screen similar to Figure 6-1 will be displayed.

Position the mouse pointer over the word **Select** in the Menu bar at the top of the screen and click the mouse button once. A list of the **Select** menu functions will appear.

Move the mouse pointer down the list until it is over the word **Patient** and click the mouse to invoke the Patient Selection window shown in Figure 6-6.

Step 3

Locate the patient named **Sally Sutherland** in the Patient Selection window. Position the mouse pointer over the patient name and double-click the mouse.

Once a patient is selected, the patient's name, age, and sex are displayed in the Title bar at the top of the window. The Catalog pane displays the message **No Documents or Images** because no documents or images have been input for Sally in the catalog.

Step 4

Because you may not have a scanner connected to your computer, you are going to import a file that has already been scanned, but not yet cataloged.

Locate and click on the Toolbar button labeled **Import.** A window of available files will open. Compare your screen to Figure 6-7.

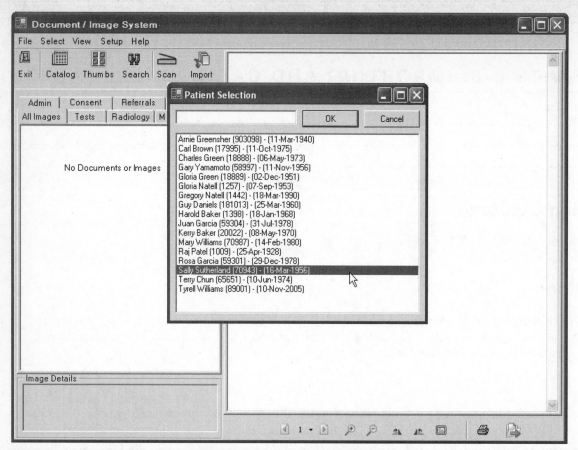

FIGURE 6-6 Selecting Sally Sutherland from the Patient Selection window.

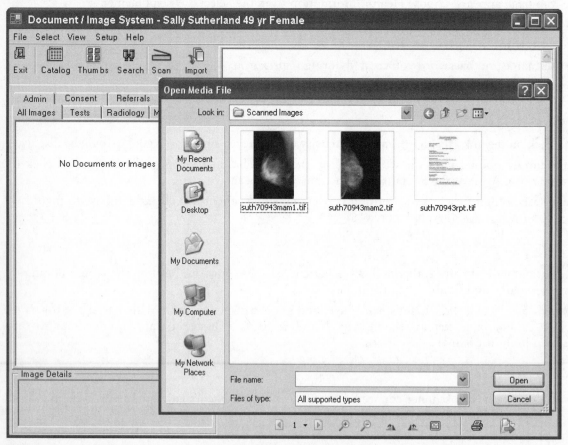

FIGURE 6-7 When you click on the **Import** icon, the Open Media File window is displayed.

Step 5

Locate and click on the thumbnail image of the document named **suth70943rpt.tif.**

Compare your screen to Figure 6-8.

Step 6

The imported file displays in the Image Viewer pane and data entry fields replace the catalog list. The fields shown in Figure 6-8 are the minimum for most document image systems. The actual fields in a catalog record will differ by software vendor or medical facility.

The image you have imported should be the radiologist's report. Note the entry **IMAGE NOT SAVED** at the top of the Catalog pane. This is a reminder to you that the report has not been saved to the patient's EHR.

The first two fields in the Catalog pane are determined automatically because the Document/Image System recognizes that you have imported the file and that you are performing a manual entry of the catalog data. Other options for these fields are **Scanned** image and **Automatic** cataloging (e.g., from a barcode.).

The Category field uses short mnemonic codes to represent longer category names, for example **HIST** for Medical/Surgical History, or RAD for Radiology.

The first field you will need to enter is the Category type. Use your mouse to click on the arrow to the right of the Category field; a drop-down list will appear. Select the code RAD, because you are cataloging a Radiology study.

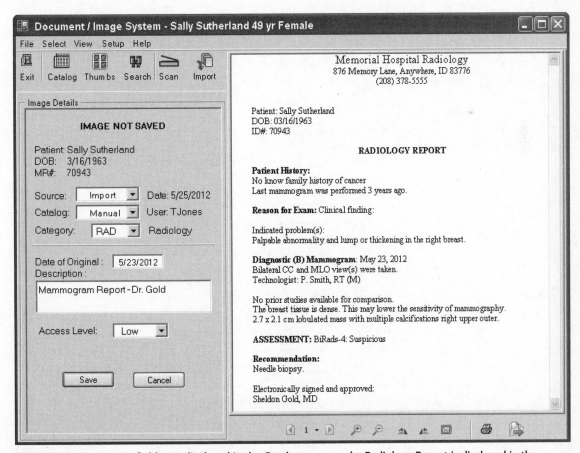

FIGURE 6-8 Data entry fields are displayed in the Catalog pane, and a Radiology Report is displayed in the Image Viewer pane.

Organization, Storage, and Management of Health Records

The next field is the date of the original document. This is used for reference purposes to locate a document by the date of the report, letter, surgery, etc. Note that the system will automatically record other dates, such as the date of the scan, the date it was cataloged, etc. These other dates are used for audit purposes.

Look at the image displayed in the Image Viewer pane and locate the date of the report; enter **May 23, 2012** in the Date of Original field in the Catalog pane.

The final field you must complete is the Description field. A portion of the description displays in the catalog list and is used by others at the healthcare facility to find the document/image. Although, the field can hold a lengthy description only the first portion of it is displayed in the catalog list; therefore, when cataloging documents and images, be sure to put the most important information at the beginning of the description. In this case, you will type **Mammogram Report-Dr. Gold.**

Compare your fields to those shown in Figure 6-8. If everything is correct, click on the button labeled **Save.**

The Catalog pane will now display your cataloged listing, as shown in Figure 6-9.

Step 7

Now catalog the corresponding diagnostic images.

On the Toolbar, locate and click the icon labeled **Import.** The Open Media File window (shown previously in Figure 6-7) will be displayed.

Click on the **first** thumbnail (the mammogram.)

The mammogram will be displayed as shown in Figure 6-10.

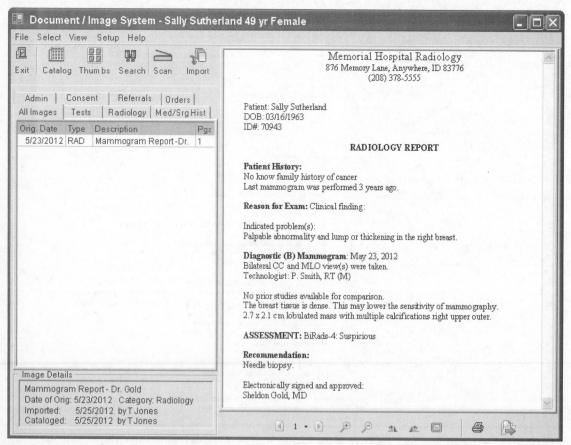

FIGURE 6-9   Cataloged mammogram report.

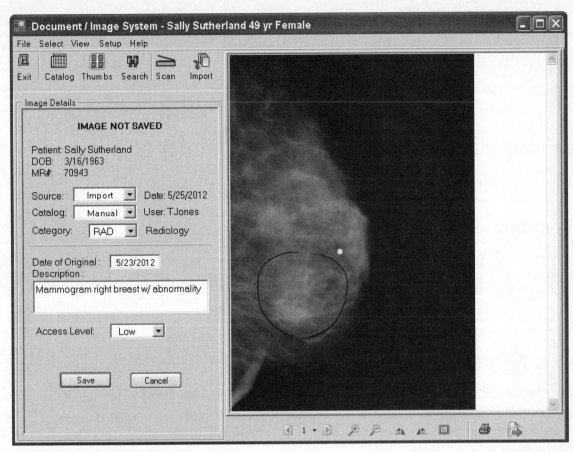

FIGURE 6-10 Cataloged mammogram image.

Step 8

Enter the cataloging data in the Catalog pane entry fields as follows:

Category: **RAD**

Date: **May 23, 2012**

Description: **Mammogram right breast w/abnormality.**

Click the button labeled **Save.**

The Catalog pane will now display two listings.

Step 9

Catalog the second diagnostic image by clicking the Toolbar icon labeled **Import.** When the Open Media File window appears, click on the **second** thumbnail (also a mammogram.)

Enter the catalog data in the Catalog pane entry fields as follows:

Category: **RAD**

Date: **May 23, 2012**

Description: **Mammogram left breast.**

Click the button labeled **Save.** The Catalog pane will now display three listings.

Activity 6-8 is concluded. You may exit and close your browser or proceed to the next activity.

ACTIVITY 6-9: RETRIEVING A SCANNED LAB REPORT

Name: _____

Date: _____

Course: _____

Learning Outcome

Explain the processes involved in document imaging.

Directions

In this exercise you will use a document image system to locate information from a recent lab report for a patient. This involves retrieving a scanned lab report and looking up a lab value. You will need access to the Internet for this exercise.

Step 1

If you are still logged in from the previous exercise proceed to Step 2; otherwise, start your web browser program.

In the address bar, type the URL listed inside the cover of your textbook and press the Enter key.

When the web page appears, choose **Health Information** from the Select a Discipline menu.

Find the picture of the *Health Information Technology and Management* textbook cover and click on it.

Click **Student Login.**

Enter the user name and password you created during registration.

Click on the button labeled **Document Imaging Exercises.**

Step 2

Locate and click on the link **Health Information Activity 6-9.** A screen similar to Figure 6-1 (see Activity 6-7) will be displayed.

Position the mouse pointer over the word **Select** in the Menu bar at the top of the screen and click the mouse button once. A list of the **Select** menu functions will appear.

Move the mouse pointer down the list until it is over the word **Patient** and click the mouse to invoke the Patient Selection window shown in Figure 6-2 (see Activity 6-7).

Select patient **Raj Patel.**

Step 3

On **February 8, 2012,** the facility received the results of a lab test performed by **Quest** laboratories. The lab report was scanned and cataloged in Raj Patel's chart.

Locate the catalog entry for this lab report and click on it to display the report.

Step 4

When the report is displayed in the Image Viewer, locate the results for the test component "Triglycerides" and write down the value on a sheet of paper with your name and the current date.

Step 5

Close your browser window and give your paper to your instructor.

ACTIVITY 6-10: ESSAY

Name: _____

Date: _____

Course: _____

Learning Outcome

Discuss the HIM responsibilities of the legal health record.

Directions

Write a one-page essay discussing the health information manager's responsibilities with the legal health record. Discuss all necessary reports that must be generated, record retention, archival and destruction, release of information, and production of legal records.

_____
_____
_____
_____
_____
_____
_____
_____
_____
_____
_____
_____
_____
_____
_____
_____
_____
_____
_____
_____
_____
_____
_____
_____
_____
_____
_____

ACTIVITY 6-11: CODE OF ETHICS PRESENTATION

Name: _____

Date: _____

Course: _____

Learning Outcome

Describe the AHIMA code of ethics.

Directions

Read the AHIMA code of ethics found on page 146 of the textbook. Create a PowerPoint presentation about the code that includes information about its values, purpose, and use and the obligations of HIM professionals.

Notes:

_____

_____

_____

_____

_____

_____

_____

_____

_____

_____

_____

_____

_____

_____

_____

_____

_____

_____

_____

_____

_____

WEBSITE RESOURCES

American Association of Healthcare Administrative Management

www.aaham.org

The American Association of Healthcare Administrative Management's mission is to be the premier professional organization in healthcare administrative management. Through a national organization and local chapters, AAHAM provides quality member services and leadership in the areas of education, communication, representation, professional standards, and certification.

American Medical Technologists

www.amt1.com

The American Medical Technologists is a nonprofit certification agency. Its certifications include medical technologists, medical lab assistants, medical administrative specialists, and allied health instructors others.

Health Intelligence Network

www.hin.com

The Health Intelligence Network website has the latest information on trends in healthcare, news analysis, publication forums, and subscription details.

HCPro, Inc.

www.hcpro.com

HCPro, Inc., is a leading provider of integrated information, education, training, and consulting products and services in the areas of healthcare regulation and compliance. HCPro provides this specialized information through a variety of products, including magazines, newsletters, books, videos, audio conferences, training handbooks, e-mail newsletters, and online courses.

Coding Institute

www.codinginstitute.com

The Coding Institute website has training materials and e-newsletters for professionals in the healthcare coding industry.

CHAPTER 7
Electronic Health Records

After completing Chapter 7 from the textbook, you should be able to:	Related Activity in the Workbook
Define electronic health records	Activity 7-1: Define an EHR
Explain why electronic health records are important	Activity 7-2: The Importance of Electronic Health Records
Discuss what forces are driving the adoption of electronic health records	Activity 7-3: Name the Forces
Describe the functional benefits derived from using an EHR	Activity 7-4: EHR Functional Benefits
Compare different forms of EHR data	Activity 7-5: Comparing EHR Data
Describe different methods of capturing and recording data	Activity 7-6: Different Methods of Capturing and Recording Data
Explain why patient visits should be documented at the point of care	Activity 7-7: Point of Care
Explain how electronic signatures work	Activity 7-8: Electronic Signatures
Describe the workflow of an office fully using EHRs	Activity 7-9: EHR Office Workflow

INTRODUCTION

The definition of an electronic health record (EHR) is the portion of a patient's medical records that is stored in a computer system as well as the functional benefits derived from having an electronic health record.

Healthcare organizations, insurers, medical schools, employers, and the U.S. government have recognized the importance of computerizing the various components of the medical record but many have differing definitions of their components. This chapter discusses the components of what should be contained in an EHR and what their role is in healthcare.

ACTIVITY 7-1: DEFINE AN EHR

Name: _____

Date: _____

Course: _____

Learning Outcome

Define electronic health records.

Directions

1. Choose from the following list three agencies and visit their websites. Review their definition of an EHR.

   a. Healthcare Information and Management Systems Society (HIMSS)
   b. National Institutes of Health
   c. American Medical Association
   d. Institute of Medicine of the National Academies
   e. Centers for Medicare and Medicaid Services

2. Write your own definition of an EHR compiled from your research of the three websites you visited. How does your definition differ from that given in the textbook or does it differ in a significant way?

   _____

   _____

   _____

   _____

   _____

   _____

   _____

   _____

3. Describe three key criteria that CPRI identified as keys for an EHR.

   1. Capture data at the point of care:

      _____

      _____

   2. Integrate data from multiple sources:

      _____

      _____

   3. Provide decision support:

      _____

      _____

ACTIVITY 7-2: THE IMPORTANCE OF ELECTRONIC HEALTH RECORDS

Name: _____

Date: _____

Course: _____

Learning Outcome

Explain why electronic health records are important.

Directions

Select three of the eight core functions of an EHR and explain how each one can play a vital role in improving healthcare today.

Health information and data	Result management
Order management	Decision support
Electronic communication and connectivity	Patient support
Administrative processes and reporting	Reporting and population health

1. Role: _____

   Importance:

   _____

   _____

   _____

   _____

2. Role: _____

   Importance:

   _____

   _____

   _____

   _____

3. Role: _____

   Importance:

   _____

   _____

   _____

   _____

ACTIVITY 7-3: NAME THE FORCES

Name: _____

Date: _____

Course: _____

Learning Outcome

Discuss what forces are driving the adoption of electronic health records.

Directions

Answer the following questions based on what you have learned in Chapter 7 of the text. You may also perform additional research to support your arguments.

1. How have the efforts of Presidents Clinton, Bush, and Obama facilitated the push for nationwide adoption of an EHR?

   _____

   _____

   _____

   _____

   _____

   _____

2. How has the information revolution of the Internet and personal computing contributed to the development and evolution of the EHR?

   _____

   _____

   _____

   _____

   _____

3. Discuss the potential effects on healthcare costs if an EHR were nationally mandated and adopted.

   _____

   _____

   _____

   _____

   _____

   _____

4. How could the quality of medical care be improved by the adoption of an EHR?

_____

_____

_____

_____

_____

_____

5. Discuss how adopting an EHR may be important in reducing costs for large government-sponsored healthcare services.

_____

_____

_____

_____

_____

_____

ACTIVITY 7-4: EHR FUNCTIONAL BENEFITS

Name: _____

Date: _____

Course: _____

Learning Outcome

Describe the functional benefits derived from using an EHR.

Directions

1. Name the three main functional benefits of using an EHR:

   a. _____

   b. _____

   c. _____

2. Describe how an EHR can aid in providing better health maintenance than traditional medical records systems:

   _____

   _____

   _____

   _____

   _____

   _____

   _____

3. Describe trend analysis.

   _____

   _____

   _____

   _____

   _____

   _____

4. How could trend analysis assist physicians in providing better quality healthcare?

   _____

   _____

   _____

   _____

   _____

5. What types of messages could automatically be delivered or triggered by an EHR?

   _____

   _____

6. Define decision support:

_____

_____

_____

_____

_____

7. Provide some examples of types of information support that an EHR can provide a physician.

_____

_____

_____

_____

_____

ACTIVITY 7-5: COMPARING EHR DATA

Name: _____

Date: _____

Course: _____

Learning Outcome

Compare different forms of EHR data.

Directions

Complete the following table. Refer to Chapter 7 of the textbook as needed.

Type of EHR Data	Digital Images	Text	Fielded
List examples of each form of data			
Is this data easily created so it can be included in an EHR? How?			
How can this data be entered into an EHR?			
How could this type of data be coded?			

1. Describe three different examples of digital data:
   a. _____
   b. _____
   c. _____

2. Discuss the methods for creating a text file and inserting it into an EHR.

   _____

   _____

   _____

   _____

   _____

ACTIVITY 7-6: DIFFERENT METHODS OF CAPTURING AND RECORDING DATA

Name: _____

Date: _____

Course: _____

Learning Outcome

Describe different methods of capturing and recording data.

Directions

Use a separate piece of paper to answer the following essay questions:

1. How would a medical practice incorporate a paper-based form and its data in an EHR?

2. Describe one way a practitioner could enter notes into an EHR.

3. Because laboratory orders and results comprise a large volume of the paper in a typical paper-based chart, how could their inclusion in an EHR assist the physician with the interpretation of this data?

4. Because many physicians still dictate a portion of the medical record, how might that dictation be incorporated into an EHR?

5. How might vital signs and a medical history questionnaire be incorporated into a patient's EHR?

6. Describe the ways in which an EHR can assist the physician in prescribing medications and documenting that information in a patient's EHR.

Notes:

_____

_____

_____

_____

ACTIVITY 7-7: POINT OF CARE

Name: _____

Date: _____

Course: _____

Learning Outcome

Explain why patient visits should be documented at the point of care.

Directions

1. Define the term point of care in terms of a medical office setting or in a hospital or clinic-based place of service.

   _____

   _____

   _____

2. You are the new medical office manager; Nurse Johnson is a new addition to your medical practice. She has never worked in an office with an EHR. Your EHR has terminals in each exam room. She frequently waits until the patient has left the office before completing her documentation and relies on her clipboard and paper notes. How do you encourage her to complete the patient's records during the visit? What do you tell her about the importance of "point of care" documentation to your medical records?

   _____

   _____

   _____

   _____

   _____

   _____

ACTIVITY 7-8: ELECTRONIC SIGNATURES

Name: _____

Date: _____

Course: _____

Learning Outcome

Explain how electronic signatures work.

Directions

Answer the following questions.

1. Define an *electronic signature*.

   _____

   _____

   _____

2. Name the three criteria needed for an electronic signature to be valid and write a definition for each criterion:

   a. _____

   b. _____

   c. _____

3. Describe how electronic signatures can be utilized.

   _____

   _____

   _____

4. How safe and secure are electronic signatures?

   _____

   _____

   _____

5. Use the Internet to research a recent breach of medical information that was stored in a computer. Give a brief synopsis of the occurrence, including how many patients were affected and if electronic signatures may have been falsely obtained.

   _____

   _____

   _____

   _____

   _____

   _____

   _____

ACTIVITY 7-9: EHR OFFICE WORKFLOW

Name: _____

Date: _____

Course: _____

Learning Outcome

Describe the workflow of an office fully using an EHR.

Directions

Review each of the following 12 workflow tasks related to using an electronic health record. Cut out the shapes below and arrange them in the order in which they would occur within a medical office that is fully using an EHR. Once you have determined the correct order, add the numbers to the table.

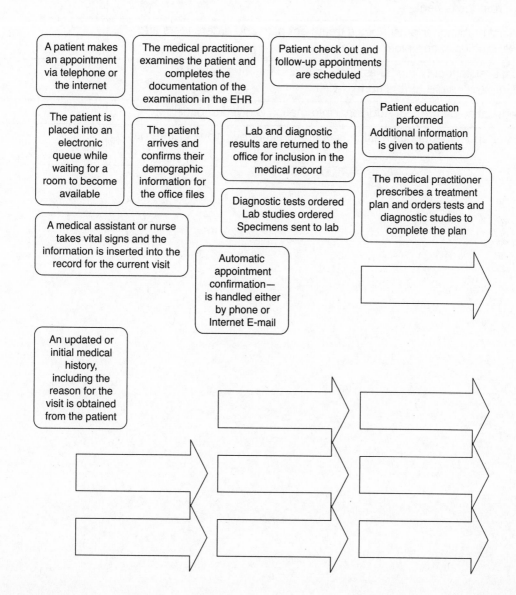

Workflow Tasks	Order in Which They Occur
The patient arrives and confirms his demographic information for the office files.	
Lab and diagnostic results are returned to the office for inclusion in the medical record.	
Diagnostic tests ordered. Lab studies ordered. Specimens sent to lab.	
Patient checkout and follow-up appointments are scheduled.	
The medical practitioner examines the patient and completes the documentation of the examination in the EHR.	
The patient is placed into an electronic queue while waiting for a room to become available.	
A patient makes an appointment via telephone or the Internet.	
An updated or initial medical history, including the reason for the visit, is obtained from the patient.	
The medical practitioner prescribes a treatment plan and orders tests and diagnostic studies to complete the plan.	
A medical assistant or nurse takes vital signs and the information is inserted into the record for the current visit.	
Patient education performed. Additional information is given to patients.	
Automatic appointment confirmation is handled either by phone or Internet e-mail.	

WEBSITE RESOURCES

Healthcare Information and Management Systems Society

www.himss.org/ASP/index.asp

The Healthcare Information and Management Systems Society (HIMSS) is the healthcare industry's membership organization exclusively focused on providing leadership for the optimal use of healthcare information technology (IT) and management systems for the betterment of healthcare.

National Institutes of Health

www.nih.gov

The National Institutes of Health (NIH), a part of the U.S. Department of Health and Human Services, is the primary federal agency for conducting and supporting medical research.

American Medical Association

www.ama-assn.org

The mission of the American Medical Association is to promote the art and science of medicine and the betterment of public health. Their core values include leadership, excellence, and integrity and ethical behavior. Through their membership and legislative efforts, they are the major force driving most modern healthcare issues as they pertain to physicians in America today.

Agency for Healthcare Research and Quality

http://healthit.ahrq.gov

The Agency for Healthcare Research and Quality (AHRQ) is the lead federal agency charged with improving the quality, safety, efficiency, and effectiveness of healthcare for all Americans. As one of 12 agencies within the Department of Health and Human Services, AHRQ supports health services research that will improve the quality of healthcare and promote evidence-based decision making.

Centers for Medicare and Medicaid Services

.ov

rs for Medicare and Medicaid Services (CMS) is the U.S. federal agency that administers Medicaid, and the Children's Health Insurance Program. It provides information for health pro- and patients. Its programs and directives affect most insurers on matters of record keeping and es pertaining to patient records.

CHAPTER 8
Additional Health Information Systems

After completing Chapter 8 from the textbook, you should be able to:	Related Activity in the Workbook
Describe departmental health record systems	Activity 8-1: Health Record Systems
Explain how departmental health record systems contribute to the EHR	Activity 8-2: How Do Different Departmental Systems Contribute to an EHR?
Discuss the factors that cause facilities to use multiple information systems	Activity 8-3: Choosing an Information System
Describe patient registration and master patient indexes	Activity 8-4: Design a Screen
Describe the workflow of electronic lab orders and results	Activity 8-5: Electronic Workflow
Describe radiology information systems	Activity 8-6: Exploring Other Information Systems
Describe workflow dictation and transcription	Activity 8-7: Follow the Flow
Explain how speech recognition works	Activity 8-8: Understanding Speech Recognition Software
Describe pharmacy, emergency department, and surgical information systems	Activity 8-6: Exploring Other Information Systems Activity 8-9: Emergency Department System Challenges
Compare implant and transplant registries	Activity 8-10: Comparing Registries
Explain the concept of clinical trials	Activity 8-11: Clinical Trials

INTRODUCTION

After reading the early chapters in the textbook one might imagine that a hospital or doctor's office has one large health record computer system. Health records can originate from many separate systems. Some of these records are imported into the EHR or into a central clinical data repository (CDR). Others are retrieved and displayed from the EHR but actually remain stored on their respective systems.

The overall health information system (HIS) includes both clinical and administrative systems. This chapter focused mainly on systems that are used by departments to perform their daily tasks and that act as the source of data for certain aspects of the EHR.

ACTIVITY 8-1: UNDERSTANDING HEALTH RECORD SYSTEMS

Name: _____

Date: _____

Course: _____

Learning Outcome

Describe departmental health record systems.

Directions

1. Complete the following diagram by writing the name of a department in each empty box. Departments include Lab, Radiology, Emergency Department, Surgery, Biomedical, Pharmacy, and Registration.

2. Next, draw lines of communication between each department that shares information or needs to share information.

3. For each department, include the types of information they may share or require from another department.

    HINT: Remember there is one central key department; place that department in the middle of the drawing! Assume the departmental systems are of an integrated system type.

4. If the system was a "best-of-breed" system, what would fit between each of the department's systems? Draw in the necessary interfaces within the information flow.

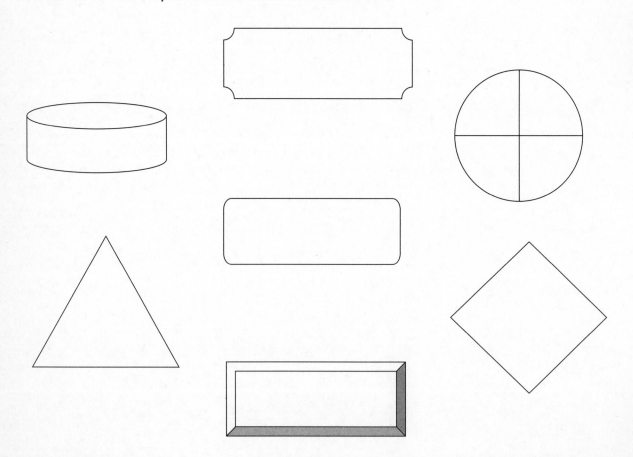

ACTIVITY 8-2: HOW DO DIFFERENT DEPARTMENTAL SYSTEMS CONTRIBUTE TO AN EHR?

Name: _____

Date: _____

Course: _____

Learning Outcome

Explain how departmental health record systems contribute to the EHR.

Directions

What elements of an EHR are contributed by each department listed below?

1. Registration:

   _____
   _____
   _____

2. Laboratory:

   _____
   _____
   _____

3. Biomedical:

   _____
   _____
   _____

4. Radiological:

   _____
   _____
   _____

5. Pharmacy:

   _____
   _____
   _____

6. Emergency department:

   _____
   _____
   _____

7. Surgery:

   _____
   _____
   _____

ACTIVITY 8-3: CHOOSING AN INFORMATION SYSTEM

Name: _____

Date: _____

Course: _____

Learning Outcome

Discuss the factors that cause facilities to use multiple information systems

Directions

Part 1

Use the following chart to brainstorm the advantages of using multiple or integrated information systems.

Advantages of Multiple Systems	Advantages of Using Integrated Systems
Disadvantages of Using Multiple Systems	Disadvantages of Using Integrated Systems

Part 2

Group activity

1. Divide into two groups; both groups are hospital department chairs.
2. Designate each group as either in favor of a best-of-breed or a single integrated system.
3. Stage a "board meeting" to discuss the advantages of each system.
4. Have a record keeper take notes for review after the meeting.
5. Have the combined boards draft a report of findings to the CFO of the hospital.

ACTIVITY 8-4: DESIGN A SCREEN

Name: _____

Date: _____

Course: _____

Learning Outcome

Describe patient registration and master patient indexes.

Directions

Design a brand new registration screen for General Memorial Hospital Patient Registration. Review Figure 8-1 on page 184 in the textbook for some ideas. You can use the space below as a design space for your rough draft. Remember to include the key elements needed for a large sized hospital registration system!

General Memorial Hospital Registration System

ACTIVITY 8-5: ELECTRONIC WORKFLOW

Name: _____

Date: _____

Course: _____

Learning Outcome

Describe the workflow of electronic lab orders and results.

Directions

Dr. Brown is the hospitalist* treating patient Betsy Smith in the ICU. He needs to order a "stat" automated cardiac enzyme test to rule out a possible cardiac event. Big City Hospital has a LIS (laboratory information system), so Dr. Brown utilizes the LIS to order the stat test. Use the diagram below to demonstrate the steps involved in getting the test ordered through the LIS.

*Note: A hospitalist is a new specialty of doctors who work only in a hospital setting.

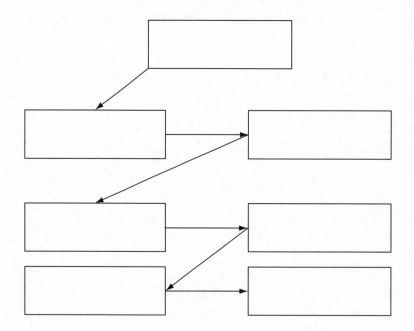

ACTIVITY 8-6: EXPLORING OTHER INFORMATION SYSTEMS

Name: _____

Date: _____

Course: _____

Learning Outcomes

Describe radiology information systems.

Describe pharmacy, emergency department, and surgical information systems.

Directions

Answer the following questions.

1. What does *DUR* stand for and what are its functions within a pharmacy system?

   _____

   _____

   _____

2. What secondary functions might a pharmacy system perform in a hospital-based pharmacy?

   _____

   _____

   _____

3. Complete the following chart to demonstrate the steps needed to place a "regular" x-ray into an EHR:

a.	
b.	
c.	
d.	

4. In an RIS, where are the digital images stored? How are they archived? What data in addition to digital images is stored in the archive?

_____

_____

_____

5. What are biomedical devices? What role might they play in the EHR?

_____

_____

_____

6. When it comes to volume of data, why might biomedical devices have more than other systems?

_____

_____

_____

7. What type of data may be stored in the medical record?

_____

_____

_____

ACTIVITY 8-7: FOLLOW THE FLOW

Name: _____

Date: _____

Course: _____

Learning Outcome

Describe workflow dictation and transcription.

Directions

Upon patient Betsy Smith's arrival in the Emergency Department, Dr. Johnson examines Ms. Smith and needs to dictate a report of the encounter. Use the following chart to document the steps that must be taken to complete the documentation of the encounter with Ms. Smith and place the report in the medical record.

Dr. Johnson examines the patient.

1. How would the incorporation of speech recognition software speed up this process? Include the possible steps in your description.

   _____

   _____

   _____

   _____

   _____

   _____

ACTIVITY 8-8: UNDERSTANDING SPEECH RECOGNITION SOFTWARE

Name: _____

Date: _____

Course: _____

Learning Outcome

Explain how speech recognition works.

Directions

1. Describe some disadvantages of a paper-based charting system and a traditional transcription system:

   _____

   _____

   _____

   _____

2. What is a phoneme and how many are there in the English language?

   _____

   _____

   _____

   _____

3. How accurate is speech recognition software and how is its accuracy affected?

   _____

   _____

   _____

   _____

4. Who is Ray Kurzweil and what are his contributions to speech recognition system development?

   _____

   _____

   _____

   _____

5. Describe a *language model* and what its function is in a speech recognition system:

   _____

   _____

   _____

   _____

6. Do an Internet search on the term "voice recognition" to discover different "free" samples of speech recognition software. Gather some information for one specific software product. If you have a personal computer, try that free software and if possible demonstrate it in your classroom.

ACTIVITY 8-9: EMERGENCY DEPARTMENT SYSTEM CHALLENGES

Name: _____

Date: _____

Course: _____

Learning Outcome

Describe pharmacy, emergency department, and surgical information systems.

Directions

1. Discuss three challenges facing emergency departments systems:

   a. _____

   b. _____

   c. _____

2. Because emergency departments need a large amount of real-time data, discuss some of the elements of emergency department care delivery that modern EHRs can provide:

   _____

   _____

   _____

3. With the emergency room (also called emergency department) system in the center of the following diagram, what other hospital systems must an emergency room EHR interface with?

```
┌──────────────┐   ┌──────────────┐   ┌──────────────┐
│              │   │              │   │              │
│              │   │              │   │              │
│              │   │              │   │              │
└──────────────┘   └──────────────┘   └──────────────┘

                   ┌──────────────┐
                   │  Emergency   │
                   │    Room      │
                   │    EHR       │
                   └──────────────┘

┌──────────────┐   ┌──────────────┐   ┌──────────────┐
│              │   │              │   │              │
│              │   │              │   │              │
│              │   │              │   │              │
└──────────────┘   └──────────────┘   └──────────────┘
```

4. Describe some types of data that may be collected and recorded in a surgical department system:

_____

_____

_____

_____

5. What other medical specialties may document information in the surgical record and what would they contribute to the record?

_____

_____

_____

6. Describe the functions of perioperative software:

_____

_____

_____

ACTIVITY 8-10: COMPARING REGISTRIES

Name: _____

Date: _____

Course: _____

Learning Outcome

Compare implant and transplant registries.

Directions

1. List some common types of implanted devices that would be in an implant registry:

   _____

   _____

   _____

   _____

2. List transplanted tissues that would be listed in a transplant registry:

   _____

   _____

   _____

3. In the event of a potential implanted device recall, what data would an implant registry maintain to help the FDA notify potential patients and physicians?

   _____

   _____

   _____

4. What types of data are kept in a transplant registry?

   _____

   _____

5. Why are "outside" network contacts needed for a transplant registry?

   _____

   _____

   _____

ACTIVITY 8-11: CLINICAL TRIALS

Name: _____

Date: _____

Course: _____

Learning Outcome

Explain the concept of clinical trials.

Directions

1. Describe the four key phases of clinical trials:

   Phase I:

   _____

   _____

   _____

   Phase II:

   _____

   _____

   _____

   Phase III:

   _____

   _____

   _____

   Phase IV:

   _____

   _____

   _____

2. In the case of a hospital EHR being used for a clinical drug trial, what considerations must be given regarding access and information contained in the EHR?

   _____

   _____

   _____

3. What kinds of data might not be tracked in a basic hospital EHR that a clinical study may need?

   _____

   _____

   _____

WEBSITE RESOURCES

Kurzweil Technology

www.kurzweiltech.com

Kurzweil Technology is a great starting point to look at the work of one of the pioneers and leaders in speech recognition technology and AI.

The Healthcare Information and Management Systems Society (HIMSS)

www.himss.org

The Healthcare Information and Management Systems Society (HIMSS) is the healthcare industry's membership organization exclusively focused on providing global leadership for the optimal use of healthcare information technology (IT) and management systems for the betterment of healthcare.

Healthcare IT News

www.healthcareitnews.com/radiology-information-systems

Healthcare IT News is a news site published in conjunction with the Healthcare Information and Management Systems Society (HIMSS).

www.biohealthmatics.com

This is a career networking portal for biotechnology and healthcare IT. This site has a wealth of information on industry leaders and an extensive knowledge base.

www.amia.org

"AMIA is dedicated to promoting the effective organization, analysis, management, and use of information in healthcare in support of patient care, public health, teaching, research, administration, and related policy."

CHAPTER 9
Healthcare Coding and Reimbursement

After completing Chapter 9 from the textbook, you should be able to:	Related Activity in the Workbook
Identify patient and insurance billing terms	Activity 9-1: Translating Insurance and Billing Terms
Name the coding standards used for billing	Activity 9-2: Naming Coding Standards
Discuss reimbursement methodologies	Activity 9-3: Professional Fee for Service vs. Institutional Service Methodology
Explain managed care	Activity 9-4: Defining Managed Care Arrangements
Compare prospective payment systems for hospitals	Activity 9-5: Comparing Prospective Payment Systems
Describe how a DRG is determined for billing purposes	Activity 9-6: Reviewing the Elements of a DRG
Explain the outpatient prospective payment system	Activity 9-7: Defining the OPPS and What Is Included in an APC
Discuss situations of healthcare fraud and abuse	Activity 9-8: Fraud and Abuse Scenarios

INTRODUCTION

The method of determining what healthcare providers should be paid for their services has changed over the years. Efforts to control spiraling healthcare costs have resulted in numerous and complex methodologies of reimbursement. Third-party payers have become involved in the payment for medical services via insurance plans. Today about 85 percent of patients have some form of health plan. The variety of health plans and reimbursement schemes used by these plans are complex. There are two basic types of fee structures, one for physicians and the other for facilities.

ACTIVITY 9-1: TRANSLATING INSURANCE AND BILLING TERMS

Name: _____

Date: _____

Course: _____

Learning Outcome

Identify patient and insurance billing terms.

Directions

Healthcare uses its own terminology for some insurance, billing, and accounting concepts. Many of these correspond to standard business and accounting terms. For each of the insurance and billing terms listed below, write the name of a similar financial concept or business document.

Claim: _____

_____

Assignment of benefits: _____

_____

Adjudication: _____

_____

Explanation of benefits or remittance advice: _____

_____

Allowed amount: _____

_____

Remittance or reimbursement: _____

_____

Adjustments: _____

_____

Coordination of benefits: _____

_____

Copay: _____

_____

Coinsurance: _____

_____

Deductible: _____

_____

Patient billing: _____

_____

ACTIVITY 9-2: NAMING CODING STANDARDS

Name: _____

Date: _____

Course: _____

Learning Outcome

Name the coding standards used for billing.

Directions

Visit the WHO, CMS, AMA, and various medical billing websites. Gather information on the various coding systems and standards and use this information to complete the following chart.

Provider Type	Coding Systems Used (ABC, ICD-9, CPT-4, HCPCS, CMS HIPAA, etc.)	Who Sets the Coding Standards for Billing? (State, federal, professional organization, etc.)
Acute care hospital		
Physician—office visit		
Skilled nursing facility		
Durable medical equipment sales		
Dental providers		
Psychiatric providers		
Chiropractic providers		

ACTIVITY 9-3: PROFESSIONAL FEE FOR SERVICE VS. INSTITUTIONAL SERVICE METHODOLOGY

Name: _____

Date: _____

Course: _____

Learning Outcome

Discuss reimbursement methodologies.

Directions

Physicians and institutional services (e.g., hospitals) have very different reimbursement methods. Complete each chart for the physician services and hospital services.

Physician Services	Hospital Services
Coding:	Coding:
Fees determined by:	Fees determined by:
Factors considered:	Factors considered:

ACTIVITY 9-4: DEFINING MANAGED CARE ARRANGEMENTS

Name: _____

Date: _____

Course: _____

Learning Outcome

Explain managed care.

Directions

Answer the following questions related to managed care. Use Chapter 9 from the textbook as needed to help you.

1. Why were managed care groups formed?

   _____

   _____

   _____

2. How does the PCP serve as a gatekeeper?

   _____

   _____

   _____

3. Discuss each of the types of HMOs. Be sure to discuss the HMO relationship with facilities and physicians.

   _____

   _____

   _____

4. Describe a capitation plan and how its reimbursement differs from an HMO.

   _____

   _____

   _____

5. How does a PPO differ from an HMO? Why might some patients be willing to pay more for the choice of a physician?

   _____

   _____

   _____

ACTIVITY 9-5: COMPARING PROSPECTIVE PAYMENT SYSTEMS

Name: _____

Date: _____

Course: _____

Learning Outcome

Compare prospective payment systems for hospitals.

Directions

Describe the differences and similarities for the various prospective payment systems (PPS). Complete each square according to the type of PPS.

IPPS Acute Care:	Outpatient PPS:	Inpatient Psychiatric Hospital:
Long-Term Care PPS:	Skilled Nursing Facility PPS:	Home Healthcare PPS:

ACTIVITY 9-6: REVIEWING THE ELEMENTS OF A DRG

Name: _____

Date: _____

Course: _____

Learning Outcome

Describe how a DRG is determined for billing purposes.

Directions

1. List the elements used to determine a DRG.

   _____

   _____

   _____

2. List 10 different DRG groups.

   _____   _____

   _____   _____

   _____   _____

   _____   _____

   _____   _____

3. List the 25 MDC DRGs in the following chart.

ACTIVITY 9-7: DEFINING THE OPPS AND WHAT IS INCLUDED IN AN APC

Name: _____

Date: _____

Course: _____

Learning Outcome

Explain the outpatient prospective payment system.

Directions

Answer the following questions. Use Chapter 9 from your textbook and visit the Centers for Medicare and Medicaid Services (CMS) website (*www.cms.gov*) to learn more about hospital outpatient PPS.

1. What is the difference between an inpatient prospective payment system (IPPS) and an outpatient prospective payment system (OPPS)?

   _____

   _____

   _____

   _____

2. How does Medicare reimburse a physician for an outpatient office visit?

   _____

   _____

   _____

   _____

3. List 10 of the top 20 Ambulatory Payment Classifications (APCs):

APC Number	APC Description

ACTIVITY 9-8: FRAUD AND ABUSE SCENARIOS

Name: _____

Date: _____

Course: _____

Learning Outcome

Discuss situations of healthcare fraud and abuse.

Directions

Before reading the following scenarios, visit the CMS website (*www.cms.gov*) and OIG website (*http://oig.hhs.gov*) to learn more about some common types of fraud and abuse. After researching these topics, review each of the following scenarios and write a brief description about the fraudulent activities each scenario depicts.

Scenario 1

Dr. Johnson visits the Shady Rest Nursing home. While there he sees Mrs. Wilson whom he recently admitted. Fourteen other patients of Dr. Johnson's have been admitted here. Upon return to his office he instructs his billing staff to submit CMS 1500s for each patient because he "saw" each patient as he walked down the halls at Shady Rest.

Scenario 2

Bob Jones comes to the ED for a laceration he sustained removing broken glass from a window at home. Dr. Johnson cleans and places a simple dressing on his wound. In his final chart he codes for a simple wound repair. CPT describes this as requiring suture or staple closure to be billed.

Scenario 3

Patient Betty Lou comes to see Super Labs for a Chem 7 lab panel. The lab bills Medicare for a calcium level, a sodium level, a potassium level test, and a glucose level test. The Chem 7 panel includes all these tests plus three more tests and reimburses at a rate of $7.50. Each of the calcium, glucose, sodium and potassium reimburses at $5.00 each. By billing these separately, Super Labs can increase reimbursement by a significant amount.

Scenario 4

While at the local shopping mall, Betty Lou stops at a kiosk where a sign advertises "Free Back Exam." The man at the kiosk sets up an appointment to see a doctor for her free appointment. Betty Lou has had back problems for years and walks a bit slowly due to her pain. When she completes her appointment, the doctor bills Medicare for the back brace that the doctor prescribes for her. Although she doesn't want or need a back brace, the doctor has written her a prescription.

Scenario 5

Bill Smith goes to his podiatrist for a routine yearly exam. Dr. Toez trims his toenails and sends him home. Dr. Toez bills Medicare for surgically removing an ingrown toenail. Dr. Toez' coders have orders to code this as a surgery due to "potential" for an ingrown, even if the doctor did not perform this procedure as a surgical procedure, just a simple trimming.

Scenario 6

Super Pills, an independent pharmacy chain, is offering their own Special Part D Medicare drug plan. Their advertising claims that they are "the only pharmacy to offer this Special Part D plan for FREE!"

WEBSITE RESOURCES

Centers for Medicare and Medicaid Services

www.cms.gov

The CMS website has pages dedicated to information on the acute inpatient PPS and outpatient PPS, including a wealth of provider and patient information for acute care facilities.

The American Hospital Directory

www.ahd.com

This website has large amounts of data on different hospital billing concepts.

ICD9 Coding.com

http://icd9coding.com

ICD9 Coding.com is a private website that offers a free ICD-9-CM and DRG classification coding look-up. It is an excellent resource for ICD-9 and DRG research.

CHAPTER 10
Healthcare Transactions and Billing

After completing Chapter 10 from the textbook, you should be able to:	Related Activity in the Workbook
Describe the billing workflow	Activity 10-1: Billing Timeline
Identify the eight types of HIPAA electronic transactions	Activity 10-2: Electronic HIPAA Transactions
Explain how electronic data interface (EDI) transactions work	Activity 10-3: Follow the Steps
Compare the differences between hospital and professional claim forms	Activity 10-4: Claims Form Diagram
Explain the functions of a clearinghouse	Activity 10-5: Diagram a Clearinghouse
Discuss the concepts of claim scrubbers, accounts receivable, and the payment floor	Activity 10-6: Complete the Accounting Pyramid

INTRODUCTION

Health insurance claims, billing, and other healthcare transactions are secondary health records. The business or billing office is one of the main departments to create and use secondary health records.

ACTIVITY 10-1: BILLING TIMELINE

Name: _____

Date: _____

Course: _____

Learning Outcome

Describe the billing workflow.

Directions

Create a billing workflow timeline for Mrs. Salvatore's office visit. Because you are the billing manager in Dr. Bonelli's office, you are responsible for every bill submitted and for maintaining each patient account. In the following exercise, list each individual step from the initial call from the patient to the receipt and closing of Mrs. Salvatore's patient account.

Account History

On August 30, 2010, Mrs. Salvatore came to Dr. Bonelli's office for an office visit and a minor procedure, incising and draining (I&D) a small abscess in her axillary region. Create a complete accounting work-flow timeline including all steps in generating a claim and obtaining reimbursement for that visit. The office visit CPT code is 99213 and I&D of the abscess is CPT code 10061. The billed charges are as follows: The office visit was $37.50 and the I&D procedure was $41.00.

ACTIVITY 10-2: ELECTRONIC HIPAA TRANSACTIONS

Name: _____

Date: _____

Course: _____

Learning Outcome

Identify the eight types of HIPAA electronic transactions.

Directions

Review the section in Chapter 10 titled "Electronic Data Interchange (EDI)." Here you will find information on the different ANSI transactions that pertain to HIPAA. Describe the types of ANSI transactions that a specific provider might use or receive. Place the specific type of ANSI transaction that each type of user submits in the "sends" box and "receives" in the appropriate box.

Sends		Receives
	Physician	
	Hospital	
	Dentist	
	Insurer	

Use: ANSI 837, 835, 276, 277, 270, 271, 820, or 834

ACTIVITY 10-3: FOLLOW THE STEPS

Name: _____

Date: _____

Course: _____

Learning Outcome

Explain how electronic data interchange (EDI) transactions work.

Directions

Explain how electronic data interface (EDI) transactions work by listing what an EDI actually does and how it works. List the major steps in the process taking a non-ANSI claim from the providers' office to actually receiving the reimbursement. Include the payer and a clearinghouse in the steps leading to reimbursement.

Claim

_____

_____

_____

_____

_____

_____

_____

_____

_____

_____

_____

_____

_____

_____

_____

Reimbursement occurs

ACTIVITY 10-4: CLAIMS FORM DIAGRAM

Name: _____

Date: _____

Course: _____

Learning Outcome

Compare the differences between hospital and professional claim forms.

Directions

1. Complete the Venn diagram to show the similarities and differences between the UB-04 and the CMS-1500 forms. Consider the key areas on each form. Who does the form represent, what information does each contain, what codes does each form use, what common types of information do the two forms share, etc.? Place that information in the center box of the diagram. Then place the unique fields information in the larger circle for each of the two forms.

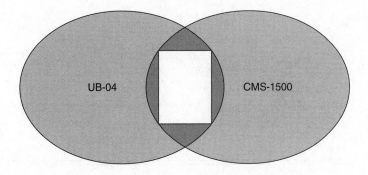

2. List some types of providers and institutions that may use the UB-04 or the CMS-1500. Remember that some providers may use both depending on their patient and situation.

CMS-1500	UB-04

ACTIVITY 10-5: DIAGRAM A CLEARINGHOUSE

Name: _____

Date: _____

Course: _____

Learning Outcome

Explain some of the additional functions of a clearinghouse.

Directions

According to HIPAA, the clearinghouse function is purely the translation of noncompliant transactions into transactions that are formatted in the manner required by HIPAA. However, "clearinghouses" may offer additional services.

Use this diagram to construct a functioning clearinghouse for Dr. Bonelli. In each box include the tasks that each "room" (i.e., function) of the clearinghouse might provide in both sending and receiving claims for Dr. Bonelli. Begin with an initial group of claims and continue until reporting and reimbursement have been completed.

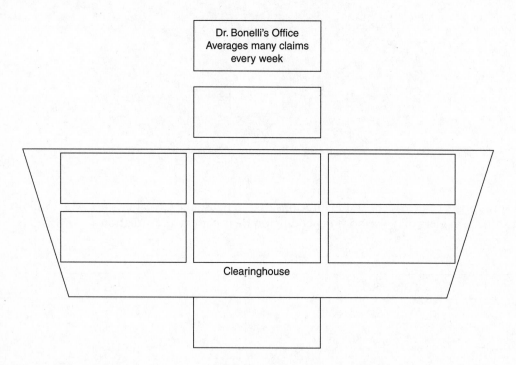

Look for some interesting information at: *www.netdoc.com/Physician-Practice-Articles/Practice-Performance/Medical-Billing-Clearinghouses, www.mpmsoft.com/EDI/clearinghouse.htm*

ACTIVITY 10-6: COMPLETE THE ACCOUNTING PYRAMID

Name: _____

Date: _____

Course: _____

Learning Outcome

Discuss the concepts of claim scrubbers, accounts receivable, and the payment floor.

Directions

In each box in the pyramid below, label the accounting and claim concepts. Place them in the appropriate order as they pertain to claims development, submission, and reimbursement. Begin with the initial claim development and the steps up to closing the account.

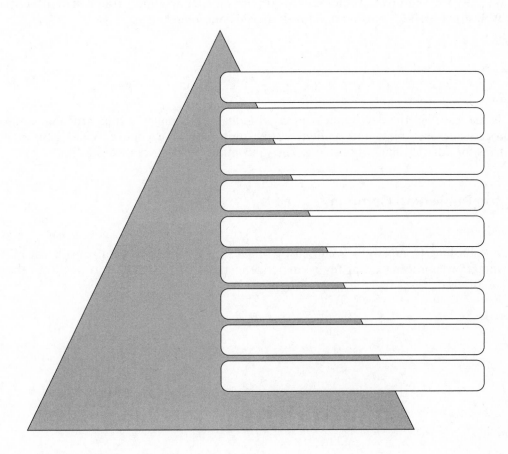

WEBSITE RESOURCES

NetDocs

www.netdoc.com

NetDocs is a physician's resource site. This page gives physicians a good idea of what a clearinghouse should provide for a practice.

MPM Soft

www.mpmsoft.com

MPM Soft is a medical practice management company. This website has an excellent primer on the basics of what a clearinghouse does.

Oregon State

www.oregon.gov

This Oregon State website provides an excellent primer on EDI activities from a state payer perspective. From this Web site, search for information on electronic data interchange.

ASC X12

www.x12.org

ASC X12 is the leader in the development of cross industry e-commerce standards that improve global business process interoperability and facilitate business information exchange. ASC X12 is organized into subcommittees for different lines of business. The subcommittee for insurance is X12n.

Washington Publishing Company

www.wpc-edi.com

Washington Publishing Company was chosen by the U.S. government to be a provider of HIPAA ANSI codes. Washington Publishing Company is an active member of ASC X12 and publishes the output of X12's subcommittees.

Health Statistics, Research, and Quality Improvement

After completing Chapter 11 from the textbook, you should be able to:	Related Activity in the Workbook
Explain why secondary health records are important	Activity 11-1: Secondary Health Record Scenarios
Describe internal and external uses for secondary data	Activity 11-2: Internal/External Activity 11-10: Additional Indexes
Discuss different types of registries	Activity 11-3: Registries
Compare the differences between an index and a registry	Activity 11-4: Comparing a Registry and an Index Activity 11-10: Additional Indexes
Discuss HEDIS and the National Hospital Quality Measures	Activity 11-5: Researching NHQM Individual Measures
Read an XML formatted file	Activity 11-6: Reading an XML File
Explain data sampling	Activity 11-7: Writing a Data Sampling Analysis Proposal
Understand healthcare statistical terms and formulas	Activity 11-8: Performing Statistical Calculations
Perform statistical calculations for *ratio*, *proportion*, *mean*, *median*, *mode*, and *range*	Activity 11-8: Performing Statistical Calculations
Describe the relationship between hospital quality measures and pay-for-performance initiatives	Activity 11-9: Defining the Road Map to Quality Improvement

INTRODUCTION

You learned in Chapter 10 about the process of creating secondary health records as claims, which are used to obtain reimbursement. In Chapter 11, you learned how claim data is also used for quality improvement purposes. Data from UB-04 and ANSI 837-I claims is used by CMS and state agencies to derive numerous healthcare statistics, including the hospital case mix index. In addition to claims, providers submit data in several other forms. Some examples are the Uniform Hospital Discharge Data Set, HEDIS, and cancer and implant registries.

ACTIVITY 11-1: SECONDARY HEALTH
RECORD SCENARIOS

Name: _____

Date: _____

Course: _____

Learning Outcome

Explain why secondary health records are important.

Directions

1. Describe in your own words what is meant by a secondary health record. You may want to review Chapters 5 and 11 of the textbook before completing this question.

   _____

   _____

   _____

   _____

   _____

   _____

   _____

   _____

   _____

2. Please provide three scenarios that demonstrate the uses of a secondary health record. For example, a secondary health record for a cancer patient is kept at Doctors' Medical Center in Atlanta. This record set details all patients treated there and specifically is used to measure the effectiveness of breast cancer treatments involving the use of chemotherapy agents in women over age 40.

   Scenario 1: _____

   _____

   _____

   _____

   Scenario 2: _____

   _____

   _____

   _____

   Scenario 3: _____

   _____

   _____

   _____

ACTIVITY 11-2: INTERNAL/EXTERNAL

Name: _____

Date: _____

Course: _____

Learning Outcome

Describe internal and external uses for secondary data.

Directions

What might a provider, hospital, Medicare carrier, private insurer, or drug company use a secondary data set for? Give some examples for each of the following types of users.

1. Dr. Juan Carlos, cardiologist:

   _____

   _____

   _____

2. Doctors' Medical Center of Atlanta:

   _____

   _____

   _____

3. Palmetto GBA Medicare carrier for California and Nevada:

   _____

   _____

   _____

4. Wellmark Blue Cross/Blue Shield of South Dakota:

   _____

   _____

   _____

5. Pfizer Pharmaceuticals:

   _____

   _____

   _____

ACTIVITY 11-3: REGISTRIES

Name: _____

Date: _____

Course: _____

Learning Outcome

Discuss different types of registries.

Directions

List three different registries a large teaching hospital may maintain. Describe each one and discuss the component data that may be contained in that registry.

1. _____
   _____
   _____
   _____
   _____
   _____
   _____
   _____
   _____

2. _____
   _____
   _____
   _____
   _____
   _____
   _____
   _____

3. _____
   _____
   _____
   _____
   _____
   _____
   _____

ACTIVITY 11-4: COMPARING A REGISTRY AND AN INDEX

Name: _____

Date: _____

Course: _____

Learning Outcome

Compare the differences between an index and a registry.

Directions

Complete the diagram below. Show the common elements between an index and a registry and the differences between them.

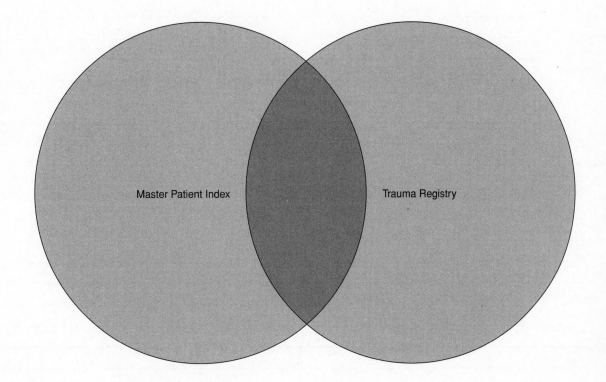

Master Patient Index

Trauma Registry

ACTIVITY 11-5: RESEARCHING NHQM INDIVIDUAL MEASURES

Name: _____

Date: _____

Course: _____

Learning Outcome

Discuss HEDIS and the National Hospital Quality Measures.

Directions

1. Visit the NCQA website (*www.ncqa.org*) to research the HEDIS measures. Select any three measures you learn about on the site, define them briefly, and discuss how a hospital may gather this information.

   1. _____
      _____
      _____

   2. _____
      _____
      _____

   3. _____
      _____
      _____

2. Visit the Quality Net website at *www.qualitynet.org* and search for the most recent *Specifications Manual for National Hospital Quality Measures* (*Specifications Manual*). Complete your research by listing each of the quality measures along with a brief description of what each measure is documenting.

   _____
   _____
   _____
   _____
   _____
   _____
   _____
   _____
   _____
   _____
   _____
   _____
   _____
   _____
   _____
   _____

ACTIVITY 11-6: READING AN XML FILE

Name: _____

Date: _____

Course: _____

Learning Outcome

Read an XML formatted file.

Directions

Review the following XML sample and then extract the data to create a simple text file. This XML file was created to extract data based on Medicare readmissions to a particular facility.

```
<ReadmissionReport>
<readmission>
<PatientName>John Smith</PatientName>
<PatientID>5467452</PatientID>
<VisitID>200807004</VisitID>
<AdmitDate>Fri, 04 Jul 2008 02:05:00</AdmitDate>
<Payor>Medicare</Payor>
<NurseStation>CCU</NurseStation>
<RoomBed>Bed 3</RoomBed>
<Service>Cardiology</Service>
<PreviousDischargeDate>Sat, 5 Jun 2008 17:21:00</PreviousDischargeDate>
</readmission>
<readmission>
<PatientID>5476542</PatientID>
<VisitID>8000200811</VisitID>
<AdmitDate>Fri, 04 Jul 2008 02:05:00</AdmitDate>
<Payor>Medicare</Payor>
<NurseStation>Station</NurseStation>
<RoomBed>Bed</RoomBed>
<Service>Cardiology</Service>
<PreviousDischargeDate>Sat, 5 Jun 2008 17:21:00-0500</PreviousDischargeDate>
</readmission>
</ReadmissionReport>
```

Notes

_____

_____

_____

ACTIVITY 11-7: WRITING A DATA SAMPLING ANALYSIS PROPOSAL

Name: _____

Date: _____

Course: _____

Learning Outcome

Explain data sampling.

Directions

Working independently or in a small group, complete a project based on brainstorming a brief proposal for a data sampling analysis for your hospital. Imagine your team is responsible for determining the effectiveness of your hospital's acute myocardial infarction (AMI) treatment programs. Write the proposal for such a report. Use the percentages deemed accurate by CMS and document the steps that you would take to compile this research.

Notes:

_____

_____

_____

_____

_____

_____

_____

_____

_____

_____

_____

_____

_____

_____

_____

_____

ACTIVITY 11-8: PERFORMING STATISTICAL CALCULATIONS

Name: _____

Date: _____

Course: _____

Learning Outcomes

Understand healthcare statistical terms and formulas.

Perform statistical calculations for *ratio*, *proportion*, *mean*, *median*, *mode*, and *range*.

Directions

Use the following formulas to solve the problems.

1. The formula to calculate a ratio is x/y = ratio. Find the ratios for the following problems:

   - In a hospital ward of Medicare and Medicaid patients, the ratio of Medicare to Medicaid patients is 3:4. If the ward contains 120 Medicaid patients, how many Medicare patients are there?

   - Dr. Johns has 30 patients, 18 of which are Medicare and 12 of which are Blue Cross patients. Dr. Jane has 20 patients, all of them either Medicare or Blue Cross. If the ratio of the Medicare to the Blue Cross patients is the same for both Dr. Johns and Dr. Jane, then Dr. Johns has how many more Blue Cross patients than Dr. Jane?

   - A special cereal mixture for newborns contains rice, wheat, and corn in the ratio of 2:3:5. If a bag of the mixture contains 3 pounds of rice, how much corn does it contain?

   - The scrub supply company sells scrub shirts in only three colors: red, blue, and green. The colors are in the ratio of 3 to 4 to 5. If the medical supply company has 20 blue scrub shirts, how many scrub shirts does it have altogether?

   - Jack and Jill went upstairs to the supply cabinets to pick saline and dextrose IV fluids. Jack picked 10 dextrose and 15 saline, and Jill picked 20 dextrose and some saline. The ratios of dextrose to saline picked by both Jack and Jill were the same. Determine how many saline Jill picked.

2. The formula to calculate a proportion is $x/(x + y)$ = proportion. Find the proportions for the following problems:

   - Jane wheeled 100 meters in her new wheelchair in 15 seconds. How long did she take to complete 1 meter?

- If 4/7 of an oxygen tank can be filled in 2 minutes, how many minutes will it take to fill the whole tank?

- An ambulance travels 125 miles in 3 hours. How far would it travel in 5 hours?

- It takes four men 6 hours to repair a leak in the hospital roof. How long will it take seven men to do the job if they work at the same rate?

- The weights of objects in the whirlpool are proportional to their weights on the floor. Suppose a 180-lb man weighs 30 lb in the whirlpool. What will a 60-lb boy weigh in the whirlpool?

3. The formula to calculate the mean is the sum of the values divided by the frequency. Find the means for the following problems:
   - Calculate the mean age of the patients in the ICU if their ages are as follows: 45, 50, 51, 60, 61, 62, 63, 51. _____
   - Calculate the mean IQ of surgeons from this list: 144, 150, 167, 139, 155, 147, 141. _____
   - Calculate the mean glucose level in all diabetics tested today: 160, 97, 150, 226, 305, 106 _____
   - Calculate the mean cost of a hospital ICU stay based on these numbers: $15,000; $7,998; $5,600; $4,257; $27,350; $11,745; $40,123 _____
   - Calculate the mean number of nurses available on the floor in the hospital on the night shift: 7, 7, 11, 4, 11, 6, 5, 11, 12, 5, 11, 7, 10, 4 _____

4. The median is the midpoint in a group of ranked values that divides the data into two equal parts. If the list of values has an even number of values, then the median is the average of the center two values; if the list has an odd number of values, then the median is the value at the center of the list. Find the median for each of the following lists of numbers:
   - 3, 7, 5, 13, 20, 23, 39, 23, 40, 23, 14, 12, 56, 23, 29 _____
   - 23, 24, 25, 35, 31, 32, 35, 33, 51, 22, 23, 34, 35 _____
   - 44, 45, 51, 50, 56, 60, 55, 45, 46, 27, 33, 57 _____
   - 3, 13, 7, 5, 21, 24, 23, 40, 23, 14, 12, 56, 24, 29, 40, 12, 40 _____
   - 3, 5, 7, 9, 11, 2, 4, 5, 23, 14, 39, 56, 28, 11, 8, 14, 11 _____

5. The mode is a value that occurs most often in the frequency distribution. Find the mode for each of the following lists of numbers:
   - 3, 7, 5, 13, 20, 23, 39, 23, 40, 23, 14, 12, 56, 23, 29 _____
   - 23, 24, 25, 35, 31, 32, 35, 33, 51, 22, 23, 34, 35 _____
   - 44, 45, 51, 50, 56, 60, 55, 45, 46, 27, 33, 57 _____
   - 3, 13, 5, 21, 24, 23, 40, 23, 14, 12, 56, 24, 29, 40, 12, 40 _____
   - 3, 5, 7, 9, 11, 2, 4, 5, 23, 14, 39, 56, 28, 11, 8, 14, 11 _____

6. Range is the measure of spread between the smallest values and the largest values in a frequency distribution. Find the range for each of the following lists of numbers:
   - 31, 32, 33, 40, 50, 51, 55 _____
   - 50, 60, 75, 76, 80, 82 _____
   - 110, 120,114, 116, 120, 160 _____
   - 80, 85, 72, 91, 45, 65, 70 _____
   - 300, 254, 300, 196, 188, 192, 300 _____

ACTIVITY 11-9: DEFINING THE ROAD MAP TO QUALITY IMPROVEMENT

Name: _____

Date: _____

Course: _____

Learning Outcome

Describe the relationship between hospital quality measures and pay-for-performance initiatives.

Directions

1. What is the Road Map to Quality Improvement?

   _____

   _____

   _____

2. What is the Road Map to Quality Measurement?

   _____

   _____

   _____

3. Create a road map to quality care. Locate the key elements along the way.

   _____

   _____

   _____

   Visit the following websites for more information:

   www.mjain.net/medicine/roadmap_for_quality_improvement.pdf. Dr. Manoj Jain, MD, MPH, is an infectious disease physician, a writer, and a national leader in healthcare quality improvement. *http://www.cms.gov/QualityInitiativesGenInfo/* Scroll to the bottom of the page, locate and click on the link to download the Road Map for Quality Measurement PDF file, the CMS web page that discusses the Hospital Quality Initiatives.

ACTIVITY 11-10: ADDITIONAL INDEXES

Name: _____

Date: _____

Course: _____

Learning Outcomes

Describe internal and external uses for secondary data.

Compare the differences between an index and a registry.

Directions

Indexes can be kept manually or in spreadsheet form if your facility does not have an electronic health record. These indexes are a collection of abstracted information utilized for statistical analyses and research purposes. These indexes are typically sorted according to their title. For example, the Disease Index is sorted by the primary diagnosis code and the Physician Index is sorted by the physician number or name.

Use Excel, Microsoft Word, or another program to create a data collection tool that includes the following fields:

Physician Name

Physician Number

Patient Last Name

Patient First Name

Patient Middle Initial

Record Number

DOB

Gender

Date & Time of Admission

Date & Time of Discharge

Service Type

Discharge Status

Principle Dx ICD-9-CM Code

Sample:

Principle Dx ICD-9-CM Code	Secondary Dx Code	3rd Dx Code	4th Dx Code	Primary Procedure Code	Secondary Procedure Code	Patient Last Name	Patient First Name	Patient Middle Initial	Record Number	DOB

Then utilize the mock patient records located in the appendix to collect and enter this data for 10 different patients.

WEBSITE RESOURCES

QualityNet

www.qualitynet.org

QualityNet's website provides healthcare quality improvement news, resources, and data reporting tools and applications used by healthcare providers and others. "QualityNet is the only CMS-approved website for secure communications and healthcare quality data exchange between quality improvement organizations (QIOs), hospitals, physician offices, nursing homes, end-stage renal disease (ESRD) networks and facilities, and data vendors."

National Committee for Quality Assurance

www.ncqa.org

The National Committee for Quality Assurance is a private not-for-profit organization dedicated to improving healthcare quality. Since its founding in 1990, NCQA has been a central figure in driving improvement throughout the healthcare system, helping to elevate the issue of healthcare quality to the top of the national agenda. From this website, click on the menu item HEDIS, and then click on the link for more information.

Centers for Medicaid and Medicare Services (CMS)

www.cms.gov

Search the CMS website for information on the hospital quality initiatives and a detailed list of resources.

Agency for Healthcare Research and Quality

www.ahrq.gov

AHRQ is a government agency tasked with reporting on healthcare issues and quality improvement.

Online Math Learning.com

www.onlinemathlearning.com/index.html

This online math learning site includes math guidelines and the formulas used in this chapter. It also serves as a resource for the student and instructor alike in math formulas for algebraic, statistics, and probability calculations.

CHAPTER 12
Management and Decision Support Systems

After completing Chapter 12 from the textbook, you should be able to:	Related Activity in the Workbook
Explain the difference between integrated and interfaced systems	Activity 12-1: Understanding Integrated and Interfaced Systems
Discuss administrative systems used for managerial support	Activity 12-2: Understanding the Components and Utilization of ADT and A/R Systems
Describe eight types of financial systems used in healthcare	Activity 12-3: General Ledger Systems
Explain different functions of human resources systems	Activity 12-4: Understanding HR Systems and Their Functions
Compare different types of patient and employee scheduling systems	Activity 12-5: Designing an OR Screen
Describe several facility maintenance systems	Activity 12-6: Facility Management Reporting Diagram
Describe different types of data collected and used by quality management	Activity 12-7: Quality Measures and Quality Management Systems Activity 12-9: Quantitative Analysis and Qualitative Analysis
Compare and contrast risk assessment and risk management	Activity 12-8: Risk Assessment and Management Team Exercise

INTRODUCTION

Healthcare facilities are complex entities and have many aspects of operation, of which nearly all are computerized. Chapter 12 introduced information systems that support healthcare operations but are not clinical records. That is not to say the systems do not contain PHI—many of them do; it is that the purpose of these systems is to support the management of the healthcare organization as opposed to being used to provide patient services.

ACTIVITY 12-1: UNDERSTANDING INTEGRATED AND INTERFACED SYSTEMS

Name: _____

Date: _____

Course: _____

Learning Outcome

Explain the difference between integrated and interfaced systems.

Directions

1. Complete the definition for each of the following terms

   An *integrated* decision support system

   _____

   _____

   An *interfaced* decision support system:

   _____

   _____

2. Diagram how each type of system interacts within a large hospital

Integrated System	Interfaced System

ACTIVITY 12-2: UNDERSTANDING THE COMPONENTS AND UTILIZATION OF ADT AND A/R SYSTEMS

Name: _____

Date: _____

Course: _____

Learning Outcome

Discuss administrative systems used for managerial support.

Directions

1. Define the components of an ADT system.

   _____

   _____

2. Define the components of an A/R system.

   _____

   _____

3. How might a hospital utilize a purchasing system to ensure they have sufficient supplies during flu season, their busiest time of the year?

   _____

   _____

4. If you were the chief financial officer for General Memorial Hospital how would you use both an ADT and your various financial information systems to make a determination about building a new Labor and Delivery suite for the hospital?

   _____

   _____

ACTIVITY 12-3: GENERAL LEDGER SYSTEMS

Name: _____

Date: _____

Course: _____

Learning Outcome

Describe eight types of financial systems used in healthcare.

Directions

For each financial system shown here, describe its function and relation to the general ledger.

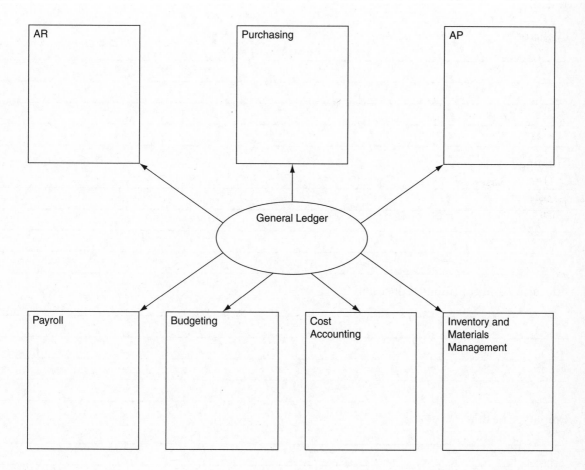

ACTIVITY 12-4: UNDERSTANDING HR SYSTEMS AND THEIR FUNCTIONS

Name: _____

Date: _____

Course: _____

Learning Outcome

Explain different functions of human resources systems.

Directions

Considering that 60 to 70 percent of a typical healthcare budget consists of personnel costs, discuss the importance of the following human resource systems and what they provide to a human relations department.

1. Evaluations

   _____

   _____

   _____

   _____

   _____

2. Training

   _____

   _____

   _____

   _____

   _____

3. Education and continuing education

   _____

   _____

   _____

   _____

   _____

4. Employee health

   _____

   _____

   _____

   _____

   _____

ACTIVITY 12-5: DESIGNING AN OR SCREEN

Name: _____

Date: _____

Course: _____

Learning Outcome

Compare different types of patient and employee scheduling systems.

Directions

1. Design an operating room schedule screen for General Memorial Hospital. The hospital has four ORs. Three are open from 0700 hours to 1900 hours; the fourth needs to be open 24 hours a day because the hospital is a Level 1 trauma center. Include such information as patient name, physician, anesthesiologist, reason for surgery, estimated time needed, OR reset time needed for cleaning and restocking of equipment, OR team, and any additional resources needed.

2. Design an OR personnel schedule to match the main OR schedule from part 1. Include a "clean nurse," a circulating nurse, an OR tech, a cleanup team and a supervising nurse for the entire OR department. If you do not have access to a computer, you may draw the schedule as a representation of the computer screen.

Note: A "clean" OR nurse is scrubbed in and maintains sterility within the operating field, whereas a "dirty" OR nurse is still scrubbed in and within sterility maintenance, but not considered sterile enough to be within the operating field.

ACTIVITY 12-6: FACILITY MANAGEMENT REPORTING DIAGRAM

Name: _____

Date: _____

Course: _____

Learning Outcome

Describe several facility maintenance systems.

Directions

Use the space below to diagram how facility departments submit information to the hospital management officer. In each department define what department personnel may need to report to the main facility officer/manager. Include the following departments for General Memorial Hospital: radiology, laboratory, biomedical, nuclear medicine, OR, central supply, fire control, and security. For additional insights visit the Joint Commission website at *www.jointcommission.org*.

ACTIVITY 12-7: QUALITY MEASURES
AND QUALITY MANAGEMENT SYSTEMS

Name: _____

Date: _____

Course: _____

Learning Outcome

Describe different types of data collected and used by quality management.

Directions

Visit the following websites, or others you find on your own, to search for information related to the types of data that is collected and used by quality management. Choose a quality measure and then, utilizing the information from your research, describe how the data might be collected in a quality management system. Could your hospital fulfill the reporting requirements from such a system?

- **Centers for Medicare and Medicaid Services (CMS)**

  www.cms.gov
- **MIDAS+**

  www.midasplus.com
- **McKesson**

  www.mckesson.com

  Investigate their information related to the InterQual software.

ACTIVITY 12-8: RISK ASSESSMENT AND MANAGEMENT TEAM EXERCISE

Name: _____

Date: _____

Course: _____

Learning Outcome

Compare and contrast risk assessment and risk management.

Directions

1. Define the following:

    Risk assessment:

    _____

    _____

    _____

    Risk management:

    _____

    _____

    _____

2. The next part of this assignment is designed as a team activity, although you may also complete it with just one other person. Ideally, divide the class into two groups. One group is the assessment team and the other is the management team. Each team should read the following scenario, and then discuss their conclusions and suggestions for examining and reducing the problem.

Scenario

General Memorial Hospital has had a number of slip and fall accidents in the hospital this year. In fact it seems like there have been more than ever, with 47 reported incidents already in the first half of the fiscal year.

   a. As a risk assessment team, what would you do to assess the problem? Is it as large as you thought or is any risk acceptable? How should the team proceed?

   b. As the management team, what recommendations would you expect the assessment team to make? Are there any additional recommendations that you may suggest? How would you complete the management portion by reducing the risk of slips and falls at General Memorial Hospital?

ACTIVITY 12-9: QUANTITATIVE ANALYSIS AND QUALITATIVE ANALYSIS

Name: _____

Date: _____

Course: _____

Learning Outcome

Describe different types of data collected and used by quality management.

Directions

Quantitative analysis is the process of checking a record to ensure the required components are present. This can be done by reviewing the record and creating a deficiency slip to distribute to those professionals who need to supply the data that is missing from the chart. Qualitative analysis is the process of confirming the documentation supports the diagnoses and treatments documented in the record. The analyst will look for incomplete or inaccurate documentation. This analysis is typically completed at the same time as the quantitative analysis.

The following are lists of the reports that are typically reviewed along with the deficiencies that should be indicated. Many EHR systems have software that partially automates this process so that the communication process with the professional who needs to supply the missing data can be monitored.

Report Type	Deficiency Type Legend
History	Signature Required
Physical	Date Required
Consultation	Time Required
OP Report	Signature and Date Required
Discharge Summary	Signature, Date and Time Required
Radiology Report	Dictation Incomplete
Pathology Report	Dictation Missing
Progress Notes	Note Incomplete
	Note Missing (Date)

In a manual system, the deficiency is recorded on paper or in a spreadsheet, and then the communication is distributed to the professional who needs to amend or correct the record. This communication can be done via e-mail or, in some instances, printouts or copies of the audit can be given to the identified personnel.

Utilize the mock patient records located in the appendix to enter this data into the following Quantitative & Qualitative Analysis form that appears on the next page. Then create a letter or e-mail to the professional who needs to make the correction or amendment.

Note: Another copy of this form appears in the Forms section of the appendix.

Quantitative & Qualitative Analysis

Analyze the assigned records for the following information.

Physician or Practitioner: _____

Record Number: _____

Patient's Name: _____

Discharge Date/Time: _____

Analysis & Date: ☐ _____

Name and record number is on each side of each form.

Indicate the appropriate deficiency type for each deficiency by placing a √ in the box in front of the deficiency type.

Report Type	Deficiency Type	
History	Signature Required	Dictation Incomplete
	Date Required	Dictation Missing
	Time Required	
Physical	Signature Required	Dictation Incomplete
	Date Required	Dictation Missing
	Time Required	
Consultation	Signature Required	Dictation Incomplete
	Date Required	Dictation Missing
	Time Required	
OP Report	Signature Required	Dictation Incomplete
	Date Required	Dictation Missing
	Time Required	
Discharge Summary/Instructions	Signature Required	Dictation Incomplete
	Date Required	Dictation Missing
	Time Required	
Radiology Report	Signature Required	Dictation Incomplete
	Date Required	Dictation Missing
	Time Required	
Pathology Report	Signature Required	Dictation Incomplete
	Date Required	Dictation Missing
	Time Required	
Progress Notes	Signature Required	Note Incomplete
	Date Required	Note Missing (Date)
	Time Required	
Other (Specify)		

WEBSITE RESOURCES

The Joint Commission

www.jointcommission.org

The Joint Commission's website includes details about many of the hospital accreditation requirements.

Health Facilities Management Magazine

www.hfmmagazine.com/hfmmagazine_app/index.jsp

The *Health Facilities Management* magazine website provides a good starting point for information on healthcare facilities management.

Appendix

FORMS

Photocopy the following forms to complete Activity 5-8: Abstracting Records.

ER Record:

Form Approved: OMB No. 0920-0278

FORM **NHAMCS-100(ED)**
(9-18-2008)

U.S. DEPARTMENT OF COMMERCE
Economics and Statistics Administration
U.S. CENSUS BUREAU
ACTING AS DATA COLLECTION AGENT FOR THE
U.S. Department of Health and Human Services
Centers for Disease Control and Prevention
National Center for Health Statistics

PATIENT RECORD NO.:

PATIENT'S NAME:

NATIONAL HOSPITAL AMBULATORY MEDICAL CARE SURVEY
2009 EMERGENCY DEPARTMENT PATIENT RECORD

Assurance of confidentiality – All information which would permit identification of an individual, a practice, or an establishment will be held confidential, will be used only by NCHS staff, contractors, and agents only when required and with necessary controls, and will not be disclosed or released to other persons without the consent of the individual or establishment in accordance with section 308(d) of the Public Health Service Act (42 USC 242m) and the Confidential Information Protection and Statistical Efficiency Act (PL-107-347).

(Provider: Detach and keep)

Please keep (X) marks inside of boxes ➔ ☒ Correct ☒ Incorrect

1. PATIENT INFORMATION

a. Date and time of visit

	Month	Day	Year	Time	a.m.	p.m.	Military
(1) Arrival			0	:			
Seen by **(2)** MD/DO/PA/NP			0	:			
(3) ED discharge			0	:			

b. ZIP Code

c. Date of birth

Month	Day	Year

d. Patient residence
1 ☐ Private residence
2 ☐ Nursing home
3 ☐ Homeless
4 ☐ Other
5 ☐ Unknown

e. Sex
1 ☐ Female
2 ☐ Male

f. Ethnicity
1 ☐ Hispanic or Latino
2 ☐ Not Hispanic or Latino

g. Race – *Mark (X) one or more.*
1 ☐ White
2 ☐ Black or African American
3 ☐ Asian
4 ☐ Native Hawaiian or Other Pacific Islander
5 ☐ American Indian or Alaska Native

h. Arrival by ambulance
1 ☐ Yes
2 ☐ No
3 ☐ Unknown

i. Expected source(s) of payment for this visit – *Mark (X) all that apply.*
1 ☐ Private insurance
2 ☐ Medicare
3 ☐ Medicaid/SCHIP
4 ☐ Worker's compensation
5 ☐ Self-pay
6 ☐ No charge/Charity
7 ☐ Other
8 ☐ Unknown

2. TRIAGE

a. Initial vital signs
(1) Temperature ☐°C ☐°F
(2) Heart rate ___ per minute
(3) Respiratory rate ___ per minute
(4) Blood pressure Systolic ___ / Diastolic ___
(5) Pulse oximetry ___ %
(6) On oxygen 1 ☐ Yes 3 ☐ Unknown 2 ☐ No
(7) Glasgow Coma Scale (3–15)

b. Triage level (1–5)
1 ☐ No triage
2 ☐ Unknown

c. Pain scale (0–10)
1 ☐ Unknown

3. PREVIOUS CARE

a. Has patient been –	Yes	No	Unknown
(1) seen in this ED within the last 72 hours?	1 ☐	2 ☐	3 ☐
(2) discharged from any hospital within the last 7 days?	1 ☐	2 ☐	3 ☐

b. How many times has patient been seen in this ED within the last 12 months? ___ 3 ☐

4. REASON FOR VISIT

a. Patient's complaint(s), symptom(s), or other reason(s) for this visit *Use patient's own words.*
(1) Most important:
(2) Other:
(3) Other:

b. Episode of care
1 ☐ Initial visit for problem
2 ☐ Follow-up visit for problem
3 ☐ Unknown

5. INJURY/POISONING/ADVERSE EFFECT

a. Is this visit related to an injury, poisoning, or adverse effect of medical treatment?
1 ☐ Yes
2 ☐ No – SKIP to item 6.

b. Is this injury/ poisoning intentional?
1 ☐ Yes, self inflicted
2 ☐ Yes, assault
3 ☐ No, unintentional
4 ☐ Unknown

c. Cause of injury, poisoning, or adverse effect – *Describe the place and events that preceded the injury, poisoning, or adverse effect (e.g., allergy to penicillin, bee sting, pedestrian hit by car driven by drunk driver, spouse beaten with fists by spouse, heroin overdose, infected shunt, etc.).*

6. PROVIDER'S DIAGNOSIS FOR THIS VISIT

a. *As specifically as possible, list diagnoses related to this visit including chronic conditions.*
(1) Primary diagnosis:
(2) Other:
(3) Other:

b. Does patient have – *Mark (X) all that apply.*
1 ☐ Cerebrovascular disease/ History of stroke
2 ☐ Congestive heart failure
3 ☐ Condition requiring dialysis
4 ☐ HIV
5 ☐ Diabetes
6 ☐ None of the above

7. DIAGNOSTIC/SCREENING SERVICES

Mark (X) all ordered or provided at this visit.
1 ☐ NONE
Blood tests:
2 ☐ CBC
3 ☐ BUN/Creatinine
4 ☐ Cardiac enzymes
5 ☐ Electrolytes
6 ☐ Glucose
7 ☐ Liver function tests
8 ☐ Arterial blood gases
9 ☐ Prothrombin time/INR
10 ☐ Blood culture
11 ☐ BAC (blood alcohol)
12 ☐ Other blood test
Other tests:
13 ☐ Cardiac monitor
14 ☐ EKG/ECG
15 ☐ HIV test
16 ☐ Influenza test
17 ☐ Pregnancy test
18 ☐ Toxicology screen
19 ☐ Urinalysis (UA)
20 ☐ Wound culture
21 ☐ Other test/service
Imaging:
22 ☐ X-ray
23 ☐ CT scan ☐ Head ☐ Other than head
24 ☐ MRI
25 ☐ Ultrasound
26 ☐ Other imaging

8. PROCEDURES

Mark (X) all provided at this visit. Exclude medications.
1 ☐ NONE
2 ☐ IV fluids
3 ☐ Cast
4 ☐ Splint or wrap
5 ☐ Suturing/Staples
6 ☐ Incision & drainage (I&D)
7 ☐ Foreign body removal
8 ☐ Nebulizer therapy
9 ☐ Bladder catheter
10 ☐ Pelvic exam
11 ☐ Central line
12 ☐ CPR
13 ☐ Endotracheal intubation
14 ☐ Other

9. MEDICATIONS & IMMUNIZATIONS

List up to 8 drugs given at this visit or prescribed at ED discharge. Include Rx and OTC drugs, immunizations, and anesthetics.

☐ NONE

	Given in ED	Rx at discharge
(1)	1 ☐	2 ☐
(2)	1 ☐	2 ☐
(3)	1 ☐	2 ☐
(4)	1 ☐	2 ☐
(5)	1 ☐	2 ☐
(6)	1 ☐	2 ☐
(7)	1 ☐	2 ☐
(8)	1 ☐	2 ☐

10. PROVIDERS	11. SERVICE LEVEL	12. VISIT DISPOSITION

10. PROVIDERS

Mark (X) all providers seen at this visit.

1 ☐ ED attending physician
2 ☐ ED resident/Intern
3 ☐ Consulting physician
4 ☐ RN/LPN
5 ☐ Nurse practitioner
6 ☐ Physician assistant
7 ☐ EMT
8 ☐ Mental health provider
9 ☐ Other

11. SERVICE LEVEL

Mark (X) that apply.

(CPT code)

1 ☐ 1 (99281)
2 ☐ 2 (99282)
3 ☐ 3 (99283)
4 ☐ 4 (99284)
5 ☐ 5 (99285)
6 ☐ Critical care (99291)
7 ☐ Unknown

12. VISIT DISPOSITION

Mark (X) all that apply.

1 ☐ No follow-up planned
2 ☐ Return if needed, PRN/appointment
3 ☐ Return/Refer to physician/clinic for FU
4 ☐ Left before medical screening exam
5 ☐ Left after medical screening exam
6 ☐ Left AMA
7 ☐ DOA
8 ☐ Died in ED
9 ☐ Transfer to psychiatric hospital
10 ☐ Transfer to other hospital

11 ☐ Admit to this hospital } *Continue with **Item 13** on reverse side.*
12 ☐ Admit to observation unit then hospitalized
13 ☐ Admit to observation unit, then discharged – *Continue with **Item 14** on reverse side.*
14 ☐ Other

2009 ED

13. HOSPITAL ADMISSION

Complete if the patient was admitted to this hospital at this ED visit. – *Mark (X) "Unknown" in each item, if efforts have been exhausted to collect the data.*

a. Admitted to:

1 ☐ Critical care unit
2 ☐ Stepdown or telemetry unit
3 ☐ Operating room
4 ☐ Mental health or detox unit
5 ☐ Cardiac catheterization lab
6 ☐ Other bed/unit
7 ☐ Unknown

c. Date and time bed was requested for hospital admission

Month	Day	Year		Time			a.m.	p.m.	Military
		0			:		☐	☐	☐

1 ☐ Unknown

d. Date and time patient actually left the ED

Month	Day	Year		Time			a.m.	p.m.	Military
		0			:		☐	☐	☐

1 ☐ Unknown

b. Admitting physician

1 ☐ Hospitalist
2 ☐ Not hospitalist
3 ☐ Unknown

e. Hospital discharge date

Month	Day	Year

1 ☐ Unknown

f. Principal hospital discharge diagnosis

1 ☐ Unknown

g. Hospital discharge status/disposition

1 ☐ Alive
2 ☐ Dead
3 ☐ Unknown

1 ☐ Home/Residence
2 ☐ Transferred
3 ☐ Other
4 ☐ Unknown

▶ *If this information is not available at time of abstraction, then complete the Hospital Admission Log.*

14. OBSERVATION UNIT STAY

a. Date and time of observation unit discharge

Month	Day	Year		Time			a.m.	p.m.	Military
					:		☐	☐	☐

1 ☐ Unknown

OP Surgery Record:

Form Approved OMB No. 0920-0334: Approval Expires 11/30/2008

FORM **NSAS-5**
(2-1-2006)

U.S. DEPARTMENT OF COMMERCE
Economics and Statistics Administration
U.S. CENSUS BUREAU
ACTING AS DATA COLLECTION AGENT FOR THE
U.S. Department of Health and Human Services
Centers for Disease Control and Prevention
National Center for Health Statistics

NATIONAL SURVEY OF AMBULATORY SURGERY

MEDICAL ABSTRACT

Notice – All information which would permit identification of an individual or an establishment will be held confidential, will be used only by persons engaged in and for the purposes of the survey, and will not be disclosed or released to other persons or used for any other purpose. Public reporting burden of this collection of information is estimated to average 12 minutes per response, including the time for reviewing instructions, searching existing data sources, gathering and maintaining the data needed, and completing and reviewing the collection of information. An agency may not conduct or sponsor, and a person is not required to respond to a collection of information unless it displays a currently valid OMB control number. Send comments regarding this burden estimate or an other aspect of this collection of information, including suggestions for reducing this burden to CDC/ATSDR Reports Clearance Officer; 1600 Clifton Road, MS D-74, Atlanta, GA 30333, ATTN: PRA (0920-0334).

A. PATIENT INFORMATION

1. Facility number

2. NSAS number and list used

3. Date of surgery
Month   Day   Year
2 0 0

4. Residence ZIP Code

B. PATIENT CHARACTERISTICS

5. Date of birth
Month   Day   Year

6. Age *(Complete only if date of birth not given)*
Units
1 ☐ Years   2 ☐ Months   3 ☐ Days

7. Sex *(Mark (X) one)*
1 ☐ Male
2 ☐ Female
3 ☐ Not stated

8. Ethnicity *(Mark (X) one)*
1 ☐ Hispanic or Latino
2 ☐ Not Hispanic or Latino
3 ☐ Not Stated

9. Race *(Mark (X) all that apply)*
1 ☐ White
2 ☐ Black or African American
3 ☐ American Indian or Alaska Native
4 ☐ Asian
5 ☐ Native Hawaiian or Other Pacific Islander
6 ☐ Other
7 ☐ Not Stated

10. Status/Disposition of Patient *(Mark (X) the appropriate box)*
1 ☐ Routine discharge to customary residence
2 ☐ Discharge to observation status
3 ☐ Discharge to post-surgical/recovery care facility
4 ☐ Admitted to hospital as inpatient
5 ☐ Surgery canceled or terminated
6 ☐ Other – *Specify*
7 ☐ Status/Disposition not stated

C. PAYMENT INFORMATION

11. Expected source of payment

	Principal	Other sources
GOVERNMENT SOURCES		
Medicare	☐	☐
If available, also note whether –		
Fee-for-service ☐		
HMO ☐		
PPO ☐		
Medicaid	☐	☐
If available, also note whether –		
Fee-for-service ☐		
HMO ☐		
PPO ☐		
TRICARE	☐	☐
Worker's compensation	☐	☐
Other government	☐	☐
If so, please specify		

	Principal	Other sources
PRIVATE INSURANCE		
Private or commercial	☐	☐
If available, also note whether –		
Fee-for-service ☐		
HMO ☐		
PPO ☐		
OTHER SOURCES		
Self pay	☐	☐
Not covered by insurance ☐		
Had no health insurance ☐		
Charity care/Write off	☐	☐
No charge	☐	☐
Other *Please specify*	☐	☐
No source of payment indicated	☐	

12. Total charges $ _____ .00   ☐ Not available

D. SURGICAL VISIT INFORMATION

13. Time

			Not available
a. Time in to operating room		a.m. p.m.	☐
b. Time surgery began		a.m. p.m.	
c. Time surgery ended		a.m. p.m.	☐
d. Time out of operating room		a.m. p.m.	☐
e. Time in to postoperative care		a.m. p.m.	☐
f. Time out of postoperative care		a.m. p.m.	☐

14. Type of anesthesia   *(Mark (X) all that apply)*
a. Topical/local .... ☐
b. IV sedation .... ☐
c. MAC (Monitored Anesthesia Care) ...... ☐
d. Regional
　　(1) Epidural .... ☐
　　(2) Spinal .... ☐
　　(3) Retrubulbar block .... ☐
　　(4) Peribulbar block .... ☐
　　(5) Block .... ☐
e. General .... ☐
f. Other – *Specify* .... ☐
g. None specified .... ☐

15. Anesthesia administered by – *(Mark (X) all that apply)*
1 ☐ Anesthesiologist
2 ☐ CRNA (Certified Registered Nurse Anesthetist)
3 ☐ Surgeon/Other physician
4 ☐ Not stated/Not specified

Please continue on the reverse side

16. FINAL DIAGNOSES (including E-code diagnoses) – Narrative description

Optional –
ICD-9-CM Codes

Principal   **1.**

Other/
Additional   **2.**

3.

4.

5.

6.

7.

17. Surgical and diagnostic procedures – Narrative description

Optional –
CPT-4 Codes

Optional –
ICD-9-CM Codes

Principal   **1.**

Other/
Additional   **2.**

3.

4.

5.

6.

☐ None

18. Symptoms present during or after surgery. *(Mark (X) all that apply)*

1 ☐ Accidental laceration, puncture or perforation
2 ☐ Airway obstruction
3 ☐ Apnea
4 ☐ Bleeding/hemorrhage
5 ☐ Blood transfusion needed
6 ☐ Cardiac arrest
7 ☐ Difficulty waking up
8 ☐ Dysrhythmia/arrhythmia
9 ☐ Embolism
10 ☐ Fainting/vasovagal syncope
11 ☐ Fistula

12 ☐ High blood pressure/hypertension
13 ☐ Hypoxia
14 ☐ Incontinence
15 ☐ Low blood pressure/hypotension
16 ☐ Malignant hyperthermia
17 ☐ Nausea
18 ☐ Peripheral site burn
19 ☐ Shock
20 ☐ Vomiting
21 ☐ Other – *Please specify*

22 ☐ None Indicated

	Yes	No	Unknown
19a. Did someone attempt to follow-up with the patient within 24 hours after the surgery?	1 ☐	2 ☐	3 ☐
b. Did they reach the patient? *If yes,*	1 ☐	2 ☐	3 ☐

(1) What was learned from this follow-up? *(Mark (X) all that apply)*
1 ☐ Patient had a question
2 ☐ Patient had no problems
3 ☐ Patient had problem(s) and –

    1 ☐ Called his/her doctor
    2 ☐ Went to the doctor
    3 ☐ Called the ambulatory surgery center
    4 ☐ Came back to the ambulatory surgery center
    5 ☐ Called the emergency department

    6 ☐ Went to an emergency department
    7 ☐ Was admitted to the hospital
    8 ☐ Other – *Please specify*

4 ☐ Nothing
5 ☐ Unknown

(2) What problem(s) did the patient mention (e.g., site drainage, temperature, pain, nausea) **?**

20. Completed by

21. Date

OFFICE USE ONLY

FR code

FORM NSAS-5 (2-1-2006)

Photocopy the following form to complete Activity 5-9: Master Patient Index.

Patient Last Name	Patient First Name	Patient Middle Initial	Record Number	Gender	Race
Address	City	State	Zip	DOB	Age

Mother's Maiden Name	SSN		Place of Birth	

Date & Time of Admission	Date & Time of Discharge	Service Provider	Type	Discharge Status

Note: This form also appears in Chapter 5, with Activity 5-9.

Photocopy the following form to complete Activity 12-9: Quantitative Analysis and Qualitative Analysis.

Quantitative & Qualitative Analysis

Analyze the assigned records for the following information. Utilize available software for chart deficiencies.

Physician or Practitioner: _____

Record Number: _____

Patient's Name: _____

Discharge Date/Time: _____

Analysis & Date: ☐ _____

Name and record number is on each side of each form.

Indicate the appropriate deficiency type for each deficiency by placing a ✓ in the box in front of the deficiency type.

Report Type	Deficiency Type	
History	Signature Required	Dictation Incomplete
	Date Required	Dictation Missing
	Time Required	
Physical	Signature Required	Dictation Incomplete
	Date Required	Dictation Missing
	Time Required	
Consultation	Signature Required	Dictation Incomplete
	Date Required	Dictation Missing
	Time Required	
OP Report	Signature Required	Dictation Incomplete
	Date Required	Dictation Missing
	Time Required	
Discharge Summary/Instructions	Signature Required	Dictation Incomplete
	Date Required	Dictation Missing
	Time Required	
Radiology Report	Signature Required	Dictation Incomplete
	Date Required	Dictation Missing
	Time Required	
Pathology Report	Signature Required	Dictation Incomplete
	Date Required	Dictation Missing
	Time Required	
Progress Notes	Signature Required	Note Incomplete
	Date Required	Note Missing (Date)
	Time Required	
Other (Specify)		

TEN PATIENT RECORDS

400032: Tomei, Marissa

410024: Richards, Rickey T.

410025: Peterson, Kira

410026: Robertson, Amy

410027: Ramsey, Lyle C.

410028: Thomas, Garrett

410030: Hall, Shelly

420781: Studabaker, Ezekiel

564930: Wilson, Nora

837155: Young, Paul

Idaho Memorial Hospital
876 Memory Lane, Anywhere, ID 83776
(208) 378-5555

Patient Name	Maiden Name		Date of Birth	Record Number	Date of Admission	Time of Admission
Tomei, Marissa	Edwards		01/20/XX	400032	03/11/XX	1800

Patient Address		SS Number	Gender	Race	Marital Status	Date of Discharge	Time of Discharge
132 N. Kings Rd Kenora, ID 83756		418-63-3652	F	AM	M	03/11/XX	1905

Patient Telephone Number	Occupation	Birthplace	Religion	Length of Stay	Room Number
208 463-3822	Architect	NJ	Prot	1	ER

Primary Insurer	Policy and Group No.	Secondary Insurer	Policy Number	Group Number
Aetna	56363302	NA	NA	NA

Guarantor Name	Guarantor Relationship	Next of Kin Name	Relationship
Tomei, Marissa	self	Tomei, Adam	spouse

Guarantor Address	Guarantor Telephone	Next of Kin Address	Telephone
132 N. Kings Rd Kenora, ID 83756	208 463-3822	132 N. Kings Rd Kenora, ID 83756	208 463-3822

Admitting Physician	Service Type	Admit Type	Admitted From	Address	Telephone
Dr. Mark Tiartrop	ER	ER	Home	132 N. Kings Rd Kenora, ID 83756	208 463-3822

Attending Physician	Attending Physician UPIN	Admission Diagnosis
Dr. Mark Tiartrop	69525	Exacerbation of low back pain

Diagnoses and Procedures

Principle Diagnoses		ICD-9-CM Code
Exacerbation of low back pain		

Secondary Diagnoses		

Principle Procedure		
Bed rest, pain control		

Secondary Procedure		

Total Charges:	$589.

Idaho Memorial Hospital
876 Memory Ln, Anywhere, ID 83776
(208) 378-5555

EMERGENCY DEPARTMENT VISIT

DATE: 03/11/xx

SUBJECTIVE: This 43-year-old black female presents to the ER complaining of severe pain in her low back. The patient notes she has had a long history of back problems somewhat over two years. She notes that she was thoroughly evaluated at University Hospital in North Hampton, New Jersey, including MRI studies and numerous other x-rays. She was diagnosed as having two slipped disks in her lower back. She notes that they were not severe enough to require surgery. She was treated with muscle relaxants and was hospitalized briefly with traction. The patient notes she has been getting along fairly well until today. Today she was in church and had a sudden sharp pain in her lower back, she notes it felt like someone hit her in the back on the right side, with pain radiating down her right leg. The patient describes lancinating pains down the lateral aspect of her right leg all the way to the foot. She notes that in the past when her back has started to hurt, she has just been able to lie down for several days. Takes Flexeril and Motrin, and gradually it improves. The patient notes that she and her husband moved to Kenora a year and a half ago. He is employed by AB&B. The patient indicates she does not have a physician in Kenora, nor has she seen a physician regarding her back pain. The patient is asking for a referral to a specialist in Anywhere. I asked the patient why she chose to come to Anywhere for medical care when she lives in Kenora and she indicates that a neighbor told her that "Idaho Regional was the best place to come for any sort of medical problem." The patient notes allergy to morphine and penicillin. She is also on Inderal 40 mg daily and Dyazide for high blood pressure. She is also requesting a referral to an internist.

OBJECTIVE: Physical examination reveals a well-developed, well-nourished, black female. She is very meticulously dressed. She is, however, wincing occasionally as she gives me this history, stating that these are muscle spasms in her lower back. Temperature is 97.8, pulse 88, respirations 16, blood pressure 112/80. Exam is limited to the low back. The patient is quite tender along the paraspinous muscles in the lumbar region. She is able to flex only about 10 degrees at the lumbar spine without experiencing pain. She moves very slowly up onto the gurney. She actually walks with a slight limp in her right leg. The patient has pain on straight leg raising of the right leg of 25 degrees. The left leg is pain free until 45 degrees. She has severe pain in the right lumbar region with elevation of the left leg at 45 degrees, however. The patient has intact deep tendon reflexes in her knees. There is an absent ankle jerk on the right side, down going Babinski's.

The patient's legs are quite thin, although I do not see any asymmetrical muscle wasting. The patient also notes there is an area of decreased sensation in the lateral aspect of her right side.

Grossly, her muscle strength is symmetrical in both lower extremities, however. No x-rays were obtained.

ASSESSMENT: Exacerbation of low back pain.

PLAN: The patient was given a pain shot as she states she needed something to relieve her pain until she can get back home to lie down. She was given 2 cc of Mepergan IM. It should be noted that the nurse observed evidence of many previous injections in the right gluteal region. The patient is instructed to rest for the next several days. She is given a refill on her Motrin 800 mg three times a day and Flexeril 10 mg tid as well. I advised the patient to follow up with a specialist in Kenora. I suggested to her that Dr. Katherine Klaus had a very good reputation as a neurosurgeon and if she is having increased problems with her back, she should have her records from New Jersey sent to Dr. Klaus's office and obtain a follow-up appointment. Additionally I suggested that she should have a medical physician in Kenora where she lives rather than in Anywhere.

Mark Tiartrop, M.D.
Mark Tiartrop, MD

MCT/ejp
03/11/xx

Idaho Memorial Hospital
876 Memory Lane, Anywhere, ID 83776
(208) 378-5555

Physician's Orders & Progress Notes

Instructions: Notate progress of case, complications, change in diagnosis, condition on discharge, & instructions to patient.

Date & Time	Orders	X	Date & Time	Progress Notes
03/11	Demerol 50 mg IM Phenergan 50 mg IM DISCHARGE INSTRUCTIONS: 1. Bed rest 2. Motrin 800 mg TID #30 3. Flexeril 10 mg TID #30 4. f/u with Dr. Katherine Klaus in Anywhere. — — — — — — — — — — *MTiartrop, MD* Mark Tiartrop, MD			DIAGNOSIS: Exacerbation of low back pain

x = only the prescribed medication may be dispensed.

Physician's Orders   Progress Notes

Idaho Memorial Hospital
876 Memory Lane, Anywhere, ID 83776
(208) 378-5555

Nursing Notes

Date: 03/11

Time	BP	T	P	R	
1800					CHIEF COMPLAINT: Lower back pain
					PTA: _____
					MENTAL STATUS: _____
					COLOR: _____
					RESPIRATIONS: _____
					ALLERGIES: MS, PCN
					MEDICATIONS: Inderal, 40 mg qd Dyazide
					ASSESSMENT:
					Hx back pain , HTN
					Presents in ER c/o lower back pain
1810	112/80	97.8	88	16	
1845					2cc Mepergan Im voc hogkhip a hyrmistern
1905					Feeling "a little better." No apparent adverse reaction to meds.
					Home with husband driving
					- - - -AHolmyerst, RN

Nursing Notes

Idaho Memorial Hospital
876 Memory Ln, Anywhere, ID 83776
(208) 378-5555

AFTER CARE PATIENT INSTRUCTIONS

NOTE: The examination and treatment you have received in the emergency department has been rendered on an emergency basis only and is not intended to be a substitute for or an effort to provide complete medical care. Your own physician (named below) will receive a copy of your records. It is important, that you check with him and immediately report any new or remaining problems, as it is impossible to recognize and treat all elements of injury or illness in a single emergency department visit. IF YOUR SYMPTOMS DO NOT IMPROVE OR YOU CANNOT REACH YOUR DOCTOR, YOU MAY RETURN TO THE EMERGENCY DEPARTMENT. MEANWHILE, FOLLOW THE INSTRUCTIONS BELOW AS INDICATED FOR YOU.

Follow-up Procedures – General Instructions
You may return to work: ____ When released by a physician,   ____ In ____ days;
     If you are free of symptoms
An emergency interpretation of X-Rays/Electrocord was provided by the Emergency Physician. A final evaluation will be made by a Radiologist or Internist. You will be contacted if additional treatment is necessary.
Some fractures (broken bones) do not show at the time of original injury, but will show themselves in 10-14 days. Please return for repeat X-Rays if you are not improving.
It is common to find additional bruises and experience greater discomfort the day after an accident. If new injuries are recognized it is important to return for further evaluation.

SUPPLEMENTAL AFTERCARE INSTRUCTIONS

__ Upper Resp. Infections	___ Wound care/ suture removal	___ Splints & Casts	__ clear Liquids	__ Hypertension
__ Strep Throat	__ Tetanus Prevention	__ Fractures	__ Diarrhea	___ Assault Information
___ Croup	__ Animal Bites	__ Ankle Sprain	__ Nausea & Vomiting	__ Other_____
__ Urinary Tract infections	__ Head injury	__ Low Back Pain	__ Eye Injury	_____

INDIVIDUAL INSTRUCTIONS

Stay at bed rest. Take Motrin and Flexeril as directed on bottles. Have your records transferred here (to Dr. Klaus) from New Jersey. Follow up with Dr. Carlton in Kenora.

PLEASE RETURN TO THE EMERGENCY ROOM
IF YOU THINK IT IS NECESSARY

I hereby Acknowledge Receipt of my Discharge Instructions and Understand them.

X   _Marisa Tomei_
_____
    Patient

– – – –_A. Holmyerst, RN_
_____
Discharge Instructions Given By

Idaho Memorial Hospital
876 Memory Lane, Anywhere, ID 83776
(208) 378-5555

Patient Name	**Maiden Name**		**Date of Birth**	**Record Number**	**Date of Admission**	**Time of Admission**
Richards, Rickey T.			11/7/xx	410024	05/15/xx	1100
Patient Address	**Social Security Number**	**Gender**	**Race**	**Marital Status**	**Date of Discharge**	**Time of Discharge**
647 Armstead Way Valley View, ID 83752	518-55-3322	M	C	S	05/15/xx	1600
Patient Telephone Number	**Occupation**		**Birthplace**	**Religion**	**Length of Stay**	**Room Number**
208 455-3245	High School Student		ID	Prot	6	OPS
Primary Insurer	**Policy and Group Number**		**Secondary Insurer**		**Policy Number**	**Group Number**
Blue Shield	56243302		NA		NA	NA
Guarantor Name	**Guarantor Relationship**		**Next of Kin Name**			**Relationship**
Richards, Mary E.	Mother		Richards, Patrick			Father
Guarantor Address	**Guarantor Telephone**		**Next of Kin Address**			**Telephone**
647 Armstead Way Valley View, ID 83752	208 455-3245		647 Armstead Way Valley View, ID 83752			208 455-3245
Admitting Physician	**Service Type**		**Admit Type**	**Admitted From**	**Address**	**Telephone**
Dr. Carl Kruger	OPS		OPS	Home	647 Armstead Way Valley View, ID 83752	208 455-3245
Attending Physician	**Attending Physician UPIN**		**Admission Diagnosis**			
Dr. Carl Kruger	89524		Open Wound Left Tibia			
Diagnoses and Procedures						
Principle Diagnoses						**ICD-9-CM Code**
Open Wound to Left Proximal Tibia with Infection						
Secondary Diagnoses						
Principle Procedure						
Irrigation w/ debridement and delayed primary closure with delayed skin flap development.						
Secondary Procedure						
Total Charges:	$2489.					

162

Idaho Memorial Hospital
876 Memory Lane, Anywhere, ID 83776
(208) 378-5555

POSTOPERATIVE REPORT

DATE OF PROCEDURE: 05/15/xx

PRE-OPERATIVE DIAGNOSIS: Open wound, left proximal tibia, secondary to hematoma and infection.

POST-OPERATIVE DIAGNOSIS: Same.

PROCEDURE: Irrigation/debridement and delayed primary closure with skin flap development.

PROCEDURE NOTES: The patient was taken to the operating room following administration of light IV sedation, the left leg was prepped and draped sterilely. The open wound, which was elliptical in nature and measured approximately 4 cm in its greatest length and was spread apart by about 1.5 to 2 cm. in its greatest width with granulating tissue in the center, was excised in total. It was extended proximally and distally to create an ellipse that could be pulled together after undermining of the skin. The skin flaps were undermined at the fascial plane allowing the tissue to be pulled together quite easily.

Once this had been accomplished the area was irrigated copiously with antibiotic-impregnated solution and then the subcutaneous tissues were approximated using 2-0 Vicryl suture. The skin was then closed and run using a 3-0 intercuticular stainless steel wire. This was followed by approximation Steri-Stips over the wire closure.

Xeroform 4 × 4's, Kerlix, and bias cut stockinet were applied in a light compressive fashion. A TED hose will be placed on the leg and the patient is going to be placed in a post-op knee immobilizer. He'll be given antibiotics intramuscularly in the recovery room and then will begin a 5-day course of prophylactic antibiotics Keflex 500 mg QID. He also is given Vicodin to take as necessary for pain and will be seen back in the office next Tuesday for follow-up and dressing change.

Carl Kruger, MD 05/16/xx 1322
_____

Carl Kruger, MD   Date   Time

CPK:mm
05/15/xx:05/18/xx
Cc: MD Office

POSTOPERATIVE REPORT

Canyon Pathology Associates
873 NW 15th Ave.
Anywhere, ID 83776

PATHOLOGY REPORT

PATIENT: Richards, Rickey T.   AGE: 15

ACCOUNT NUMBER: 8246729   HOSPITAL NUMBER: 789456   DATE: 05/15/xx

SNOP NO: DOCTOR: Carl Kruger

PROCEDURE: Closure of Incision, Left Tibia Tissue, Non-Union

GROSS FINDINGS: The specimen consists of a wedge of skin and subcutaneous tissue that is up to 5.5 $\times$ 1.9 $\times$ 1.1 cm. The surface shows an ulcerated, granular, pink-tan, ovoid area up to 2.2 $\times$ 1.0 cm. Representative sections through this region are processed. Also included are two, rubbery, pink-tan soft pieces of tissue that are up to 1.2 cm. long. They are up to 1.2 cm. across. Sections are also included.

MICROSCOPIC FINDINGS: Skin surface is ulcerated and covered by neutrocytic exudate and debris. Subjacent granulation tissue is heavily infiltrated by acute and chronic inflammatory cells. There is increased vascularity and marked fibrous proliferation. Fibroinflammatory process extends through the full thickness of the skin piece. Margins of the ulcer are lined with hyperplastic, well-differentiated, stratified, squamous epithelium. Other pieces of adipose tissue and connective tissue also show reactive fibrosis and chronic inflammation.

PATOLOGICAL FINDINGS: Ulceration with severe acute and chronic exudation, skin and subcutaneous tissues, secondary closure of incision, region of left tibia.
Reactive fibrosis and chronic inflammation, consistent with scar formation, secondary closure of incision, region of left tibia.

M.B. Simmonds, MD 05/18/xx 0824

Pathologist Signature   Date   Time

PATHOLOGY REPORT

Idaho Memorial Hospital
876 Memory Lane, Anywhere, ID 83776
(208) 378-5555

Operating Room
Physical Assessment Data

Date: 05/15/xx				OR # 5

Operative Checklist

	Yes	No	NA
1. Identification Band Correct	_x_	___	___
2. Lab Reports on Chart	_x_	___	___
3. Surgical Consent Signed	_x_	___	___
4. Consent in Agreement with Scheduled Procedure	_x_	___	___
5. Allergies Noted on Chart	_x_	___	___
6. Confirmation of Surgical Site and Side By patient response	_x_	___	___

General Appearance

Pre Operative		Post Operative
_x_ Good Color – Skin Intact		___
___ Adequate Prep		___
___ Flushed		___
___ Pale		_x_
___ Cyanotic		___
___ Jaundiced		___
___ Diaphoretic		___
___ Rash		___
___ Bruise		___
___ Reddened Area		___
___ Mottled		___

Observed Behavior

_x_ Cooperative	___ Restless
___ Crying	___ Resistive
___ Withdrawn	___ Combative
___ Talkative	___ Other

Post Operative Level of Consciousness

___ Alert	___ Non Responsive
_x_ Drowsy	___ Other
_x_ Responsive	

Cardiac Monitor _____ O$_2$ _____

IV: Hep Lock

Comments: Alert male to prep room via cart with rails up. Positioned et prepped by J. Mort, RN. RN at side during procedure. Tolerated

Procedure. TOO PS in stable condition.

Signature: J. Mort, RN Date: 05/15/xx Time: 1410

Time	O$_2$ SAT	BP	PULSE	INIT.
10	97	122 / 55	52	JAM
15	95	137 / 52	63	JAM
25	95	138 / 56	58	JAM
35	95	129 / 59	59	JAM
45	93	123 / 59	48	JAM
300	94	120 / 59	65	JAM

Medications:

Drug	Dose	Method	Time	By Whom				
Demerol	50 mgml	IVP	1410	J.Mort, RN		/		
Versed	1/2 mgml	IVP	1415	J.Mort, RN		/		
Versed	2 mgml	IVP	1423	C.Kruger, MD		/		
1% Xylocaine with EP			1423	C.Kruger, MD		/		

Operating Room Physical Assessment Data

Idaho Memorial Hospital
876 Memory Lane, Anywhere, ID 83776
(208) 378-5555

Physician's Orders & Progress Notes

Instructions: Notate progress of case, complications, change in diagnosis, condition on discharge, & instructions to patient.

Date & Time	Orders	X	Date & Time	Progress Notes

05/14/xx 1205	OP
	NPO
	Prep L Leg
	
	Delayed closure w/ flap rotation
	   L prox tibia
	   C. Kruger, MD
			05/14/xx 1205	Infected hematoma s/p tibia
				Recommended for OP I& w/DPC.
				   C. Kruger, MD

05/15/xx 1510	Post-OP
	1. V.S. Routine
	2. DC when stable
	3. Kelzol i gm IM Now
	4. Rx Keflex 500 mg
	   #20
	   Sig: i po qid
	
	   Rx Vicodin – #18
	   Sig: i po qid
	
	5. TED hose
	6. RTO next Tues
	7. Post-OP knee splint
	   C. Kruger, MD
			05/15/xx 1520	Post-op report dictated.
				   C. Kruger, MD

x = only the prescribed medication may be dispensed.

Physician's Orders   Progress Notes

Idaho Memorial Hospital
876 Memory Lane, Anywhere, ID 83776
(208) 378-5555

Operative Consent

Patient: __Richards, Rickey T.__ _____ Age: __15__ _____

Date: __05/15/xx__ _____ Time: __1135__ _____ AM ~~PM~~ Place: Idaho Memorial Hospital

1. I herby authorize Dr. __Carl Kruger, MD__ _____ and whomever he may designate as his/her assistants, to perform

   upon __Rickey Richards_____, the following operations: _Delayed closure tibia wound with flap rotation_
   (State name of patient or "myself")
   and if any unforeseen complication in the course of the operation, calling on his judgment for procedures in addition to, or different from, those now contemplated, I further request and authorize him to do whatever he deem advisable to correct the complication.

2. The nature and purpose of the operation, possible alternative methods of treatment, the risks involved, and the possibility of complications have been explained to me. I acknowledge that no guarantee or assurance has been made as to the results that may be obtained.

3. I consent to the administration of anesthesia, and to the use of such anesthetics as the attending physician, anesthesiologist, an the hospital staff may deem advisable. I understand that all anesthetics involve risks or complications, serious injury or rarely, death from both known and unknown causes, and that no guarantees have been made as to the results of the anesthetic.

4. I consent to the disposal, by authorities of Idaho Memorial Hospital of any tissues or parts which may have been removed.

5. For the purpose of advancing medical and nursing education, I consent to the admittance of these personnel into the operating room.

My signature certifies that I have read and fully understand the above consent to operation, that the explanations therein referred to where made and that all blanks for completion were filled in and if inapplicable paragraphs, if any, where stricken before I signed.

See Below

_____
Signature of Patient
xxxxxxxxxxxxxxxxxxxx

_____
Signature of Patient' Husband or Wife

When the patient is a minor or incompetent to give consent:

Patrick Richards
_____
Signature of person authorized to consent for patient

Father
_____
Relationship to Patient

Melissa Clark, RN		Carl Kruger, MD	05/15/xx	1135 AM
Witness		Surgeon	Date	Time

In accordance with the Nursing Practice Act this consent must be completed by
the Surgeon and Patient prior to the operative procedure.

Idaho Memorial Hospital
876 Memory Lane, Anywhere, ID 83776
(208) 378-5555

Operative Nursing Notes

Date: Time: Pre-Op Diagnosis: Delayed Closure Tibia w/ Flap Rotation

Time	BP	T	P	R	Nursing Notes:
1208	115/70	97.4	62	12	OPS – Pre op teaching done. Pre op pre tx L leg shave & Betadine scrub for 10 minutes.
					Butterfly hep-lock started on L hand w/ hep flush.
1505					Patient taken to recovery in cart with side rails up. Patient awake, oriented ×3. Dr. takes
					Patient & father to discuss treatment regiment.
1520					DC'd Hep lock from L hand, donned ted hose on L leg over dressing, dressing dry, intact
					w/o drainage. CNS check good, pedal pulses bilateral strong. Can feel toes bilateral brisk.
1525					Dr. order received for Kefzol 1 gm RUOQ per Dr. Kruger.
1535					Tolerating fluids well, Knee splint to L leg.
1600	124/80		54	12	Father and patient both verbalizing understanding of discharge instructions. Took patient.
					In wheelchair from OPS to car for father to drive home.
					Jessica Mort, RN

Operative Nursing Notes

Idaho Memorial Hospital
876 Memory Lane, Anywhere, ID 83776
(208) 378-5555

Outpatient Surgery Discharge Instructions

FOR PATIENTS WHO HAVE HAD GENERAL ANESTHESIA, REGIONAL ANESTHESIA OR ANY TYPE OF SEDATION:

1. For the rest of today, the patient may look as if he/she has a slight fever; face might be red, and skin might feel warm and sweaty. The medication given before surgery usually causes this to happen.

2. The medicine which was used to put the patient to sleep will be acting in the patient's body for the next twenty-four (24) hours, so the patient might feel a little sleepy; this feeling will slowly wear off. Because the medicine is still in the patient's system, for the next twenty-four hours the adult patient should not:
   A. drive a car, operate machinery, or power tools,
   B. drink any alcoholic drinks (not even beer), or
   C. make any important decision, such as sign important papers.

3. The patient may have some pain. A prescription for pain may be given by the doctor. This should be taken as directed.; and if it does not decrease the pain, contact the patient's doctor. If the doctor does not prescribe anything for pain, the patient may take a non-prescription, non-aspirin pain medication which can be purchased at the drugstore. Please follow the directions on the label.

4. The patient may eat anything, but it is better to start with liquids; such as, water or juice, then soup and crackers, and gradually work up to solid foods. Babies may be fed their milk as soon as they are hungry.

5. The patient is not expected to have any fever; but if the patient does feel warm after today, take his/her temperature. If the temperature is 101 degrees, or higher call the patient's doctor.

6. We strongly suggest that a responsible adult be with the patient for the rest of the day and also during the night for the patient's protection and safety.

7. If any questions arise, call the patient's doctor. If unable to reach the patient's doctor, please feel free to call out-patient surgery. During the day (5 am – 5 pm) Monday through Friday, you may call 208-322-7575. At night or on weekends, call the Emergency Department at 208-322-7570.

Jessica Mort, RN	05/15/xx	1600	Rickey Richards	05/15/xx	1602
Nurse Signature	Date	Time	Patient Signature	Date	Time

8. The patient has an appintment with ___Dr. Kruger_____

   Date: ___Tuesday_____   Time: ___1600_____

9. Call Doctor _____ to make an appointment.

   Special Instructions: Maintain dressing and ted hose stocking until you see Dr Kruger next Tuesday. Keep dressing dry. 2. Maintain knee splint on left leg. 3. May walk weight bearing tomorrow. 4. Call Doctor if you have any problems.

Jessica Mort, RN	05/15/xx	1605	Patrick Richards	05/15/xx	1606
Nurse Signature	Date	Time	Patient Signature	Date	Time

Outpatient Surgery Discharge Instructions

Idaho Memorial Hospital
876 Memory Lane, Anywhere, ID 83776
(208) 378-5555

Patient Name	Maiden Name		Date of Birth	Record Number	Date of Admission	Time of Admission
Peterson, Kira.	Peterson		11/7/xx	410025	12/15/xx	1455

Patient Address	Social Security No.	Gender	Race	Marital Status	Date of Discharge	Time of Discharge
3127 Snowflake Way Valley View, ID 83752	518-45-3698	F	C	S	12/15/xx	2015

Patient Telephone Number	Occupation	Birthplace	Religion	Length of Stay	Room Number
208 342-3420	Jr. High School Student	ID	Prot	1	ER

Primary Insurer	Policy and Group Number	Secondary Insurer	Policy Number	Group Number
Aetna	36843302	NA	NA	NA

Guarantor Name	Guarantor Relationship	Next of Kin Name	Relationship
Peterson, Mary A.	Mother	Peterson, Mike T.	Father

Guarantor Address	Guarantor Telephone	Next of Kin Address	Telephone
3127 Snowflake Way Valley View, ID 83752	208 342-3420	3127 Snowflake Way Valley View, ID 83752	208 342-3420

Admitting Physician	Service Type	Admit Type	Admitted From	Address	Telephone
Dr. Patrick B. Manwise	ER	ER	Home	3127 Snowflake Way Valley View, ID 83752	208 342-3420

Attending Physician	Attending Physician UPIN	Admission Diagnosis
Dr. Patrick B. Manwise	83604	Probable viral guteritis

Diagnoses and Procedures

Principle Diagnoses	ICD-9-CM Code
Viral Guteritis	

Secondary Diagnoses	

Principle Procedure	
Heplock, Tylenol for Fever	

Secondary Procedure	

Total Charges:	$1289.

Idaho Memorial Hospital
876 Memory Lane, Anywhere, ID 83776
(208) 378-5555

HISTORY AND PHYSICAL

DATE: 12/15/xx

PRESENT ILLNESS: 12 yo female w/N&V. Sudden onset at 4:00 am. One loose stool. Slight dysuria & diffuse myalgia. Some aranysy abd pain. No sore throat or ear ache

EXAM: Chest clear
Abd – soft without masses or tenderness. BS active.

LABS:
UA-3-8
WBC's, no proteinuria, 1+ electrolytes
CBC-WBC 8700 with 88seg 6 bands

1. Tigan 400 mg rectally q6h prn–nausea
2. Cipro 500 mg BID #4

TREATMENT ORDERS:
CBC
U/A
RL-1000 cc
Compazine 10 mg IV
Ceftriaxone 1gm IV
Urine C&S

DIAGNOSIS:
Probable viral guteritis
R/O pyelonephritis

DISCHARGE INSTRUCTIONS
Call in 48 hrs for result of urine culture.
Notify if unable to hold down meds or fluids

Patrick B. Manwise, M.D.
Patrick Manwise, MD

SEC: pm
12/15/xx
cc: MD Office

Idaho Memorial Hospital
876 Memory Lane, Anywhere, ID 83776
(208) 378-5555

Nursing Notes

Date: 12/15

Time	BP	T	P	R	
1455					CHIEF COMPLAINT: Fever, emesis, Vertigo —V. Branson, LPN
					ALLERGIES: NKA
					MEDICATIONS: None
					PMH: Strep throat
					ASSESSMENT:
					Pt. awoke @ 0430 AM with N&V. Unable to lie supine due to abd spasms.
					Febrile. Has cont to experience emesis ×8 since onset. c/o vertigo. Unable to eat
					or drink. Last BM @ 8 am – normal. Mid-abdominal tenderness noted.
1455	114/77	101.7	156	20	
	116/74	ok	127	20	
	112/63		159		
1710					L R – 1000 22 gm @ ® arm - - -LF
1715					Compazine 10 mg IV - - -LF
1720					Increase Rocephin 1gm IVP - - -CS
1740					No adverse reaction obtained relief of Nausea with med.
1830	122/70	101.9	120	18	Tylenol tabs ii po —AW
					Feeling much better LR 600 cc in
1930		101.9			
2000					Child smiling & conversational._LR 900cc urine – Going home
2015		101.8			With IV site hep locked in case she needs to return. Mother to
					Watch temp & treat with Tylenol. - - -V. Branson, LPN

Nursing Notes

Idaho Memorial Hospital
876 Memory Lane, Anywhere, ID 83776
(208) 378-5555

CHILDRENS TYLENOL (ACETAMINOPHEN) AND ASPIRIN DOSAGE RECOMMENDATIONS

AGE GROUP	0–3 MONTHS	4–11 MONTHS	12–23 MONTHS	2–3 YEARS	4–5 YEARS	6–8 YEARS	9–10 YEARS	11–12 YEARS
WEIGHT (LBS)	6–11	12–17	18–23	24–35	36–47	48–59	60–71	72–95
DOSE OF TYLENOL (IN MILLIGRAMS)	40	80	120	160	240	320	400	480
DROPS (80 MG/0.8 ML) DROPPERFULS	1/2	1	1 ½	2	3	4	5	–
ELIXIR (160 MG/5 ML) TEASPOONFULS	–	1/4	3/4	1	1½	2	2½	3
BABY' ASPIRIN CHEWABLE (81 MG)	–	–	1–1½	2	3	4	5	6–8
ASPIRIN ADULT TABLETS (325 MG)	–	–	–	1/2	1/2–1	1	1–1½	1½–2

NOTE: ASPIRIN IS NOT RECOMMENDED FOR CHILDREN UNDER 16 YRS. WITH FEVER DUE TO CHICKEN POX, FLU, OR VIRAL ILLNESS

Check the temperature at least every 4 hours.
Use Tylenol or aspirin every 4 hours if temp. is over 100 degrees

FEVER: DO NOT USE ICE WATER OR ALCOHOL SPONGE BATH

Fever can be reduced by undressing the child in a 70-degree room.
Do not bundle up a child who shivers and feels a chill as this will only raise the body temperature.
Offer the child clear fluids as often as he will take them (Gatorade, fruit juices, popsicles, soft drinks).
Do not force him to take solid foods as appetite is often decreased.
A child with a history of fever seizures should be treated vigorously with above measures at the onset of a fever

Idaho Memorial Hospital
876 Memory Lane, Anywhere, ID 83776
(208) 378-5555

AFTER CARE PATIENT INSTRUCTIONS

NOTE: The examination and treatment you have received in the emergency department has been rendered on an emergency basis only and is not intended to be a substitute for, or to provide complete medical care. Your own physician (named below) will receive a copy of your records. It is important, that you check with him/her and immediately report any new or remaining problems, as it is impossible to recognize and treat all elements of injury or illness in a single emergency department visit.

IF YOUR SYMPTOMS DO NOT IMPROVE OR YOU CANNOT REACH YOUR DOCTOR, YOU MAY RETURN TO THE EMERGENCY DEPARTMENT. MEANWHILE, FOLLOW THE INSTRUCTIONS BELOW AS INDICATED FOR YOU.

<u>Follow-up Procedures</u> – General Instructions

You may return to work: ____ When released by a physician, _____ In _#___ days, or ___ If you are free of symptoms.

An emergency interpretation of X-Rays was provided by the Emergency Physician. A final evaluation will be made by a Radiologist or Internist. You will be contacted if additional treatment is necessary.

Some fractures (broken bones) do not show at the time of original injury, but will show themselves in 10–14 days. Please return for repeat X-Rays if you are not improving.

It is common to find additional bruises and experience greater discomfort the day after an accident. If new injuries are recognized it is important to return for further evaluation.

SUPPLEMENTAL AFTERCARE INSTRUCTIONS

__Croup	__Animal Bites	__Ankle Sprain	__Clear Liquids	__Hypertension
__Strep Throat	__Head injury	__Fractures	__Diarrhea	__Assault Information
__Upper Respiratory Infections	__Tetanus Prevention	__Splints & Casts	__Nausea & Vomiting	__Other_____
__Urinary Tract infections	__Wound care/ suture removal	__Low Back Pain	__Eye Injury	_____

INDIVIDUAL INSTRUCTIONS

Call in 48 hours for Result of urine culture – notify Dr Baker if unable to hold medication & fluids down. Remove Heparin lock after 24 hours if not needed for readmission. Use Tylenol to control fever.

PLEASE RETURN TO THE EMERGENCY ROOM IF YOU THINK IT IS NECESSARY

I hereby Acknowledge Receipt of my Discharge Instructions and Understand them.

X ___Mrs. W. Peterson_____Mother_____

    Patient signature   Relationship to patient

– – – – – V. Branson, LPN

Discharge Instructions Given By

Idaho Memorial Hospital
876 Memory Lane, Anywhere, ID 83776
(208) 378-5555

Patient Name	Maiden Name		Date of Birth	Record Number	Date of Admission	Time of Admission
Robertson, Amy	Roe		11/7/xx	410026	07/23/xx	1100
		Gender	Race	Marital Status	Date of Discharge	Time of Discharge
Patient Address	Social Security No.	F	C	D	07/23/xx	1420
1604 E Parent Loop Valley View, ID 83752	519-53-4478					
Patient Telephone Number	Occupation		Birthplace	Religion	Length of Stay	Room Number
208 431-3257	High School Teacher		ID	Prot	1	ER
Primary Insurer	Policy and Group No.		Secondary Insurer		Policy Number	Group Number
UHC	692435562		NA		NA	NA
Guarantor Name	Guarantor Relationship		Next of Kin Name			Relationship
Squires, Ann	Mother		Squires, Darrell			Father
Guarantor Address	Guarantor Telephone		Next of Kin Address			Telephone
1604 E Cherry Ln Valley View, ID 83752	208 455-9874		1604 E. cherry Ln Valley View, ID 83752			208 455-9874
Admitting Physician	Service Type		Admit Type	Admitted From	Address	Telephone
Dr. Carl Kruger	ER		ER	Home	1604 E Parent Loop Valley View, ID 83752	208 431-3257
Attending Physician	Attending Physician UPIN		Admission Diagnosis			
Dr. Carl Kruger	89524		Blood in stool last night- Hx hemorrhoids			
Diagnoses and Procedures						
Principle Diagnoses						ICD-9-CM Code
Hemorrhoids						
Secondary Diagnoses						
Principle Procedure						
CBC drawn						
Secondary Procedure						
Total Charges:	$959.					

Idaho Memorial Hospital
876 Memory Lane, Anywhere, ID 83776
(208) 378-5555

HISTORY AND PHYSICAL

DATE: 07/23/xx

This patient is a 32-year-old female who presents to the emergency department for evaluation of rectal bleeding. The patient has been constipated recently and wondered if she might have ruptured a hemorrhoid. She has had a history of constipation and hemorrhoids in the past. However, she states that she has not been aware of hemorrhoidal symptoms recently and after passing perhaps a cup of blood with her stool last night she noted that the stool appeared dark, almost blackish in color. Also, the stool was not particularly constipated last night. She moved her bowels this morning and they were not black and she had no further bleeding. The patient did not initially complain of any lightheadedness on standing. However, when specifically questioned she thinks that perhaps she may have had such symptoms to a slight degree recently. She has not had any rectal bleeding or any dark stools in many months. She tells me that as a teenager she was told one time that she had a touch of ulcerative colitis. She has been followed every 2 years with sigmoidoscopy and/or air contrast barium enema to follow her for this problem. They have found no evidence of recurrence. Her last test was, I believe, just last year. Her home is in Wagner, Oklahoma, but she will not be returning there for about a month.

Objectively the patient is bright and alert and in no acute distress. Her color is good. Orthostatic vital signs were taken and showed no orthostatic hypotension.

Carl Kruger, MD
_____
Dr. Carl J. Kruger

CJK:pm
07/23/xx
cc: MD Office

Idaho Memorial Hospital
876 Memory Lane, Anywhere, ID 83776
(208) 378-5555

Nursing Notes

Date: 07/23/xx

Time	BP	T	P	R	
					CHIEF COMPLAINT: Blood in stool last night- Hx hemorrhoids
					- - - -V. Caldwell, LPN
					ALLERGIES: NKA
					MEDICATIONS: None
					ASSESSMENT: Hemorrhoids
					Last evening @ 6 pm pt. has some mucous et blood in stool –
					Pt did take a laxative earlier, because of constipation.
					Pt states has had hemorrhoid problems in the past
					Pt states she did have some black color in stool
					no BM's since
1115	131/88	98.9	82	18	
	138/92		101		CBC drawn
					- - - -V. Caldwell, LPN

Nursing Notes

Idaho Memorial Hospital
876 Memory Lane, Anywhere, ID 83776
(208) 378-5555

AFTER CARE PATIENT INSTRUCTIONS

NOTE: The examination and treatment you have received in the emergency department has been rendered on an emergency basis only and is not intended to be a substitute for, or to provide complete medical care. Your own physician (named below) will receive a copy of your records. It is important, that you check with him/her and immediately report any new or remaining problems, as it is impossible to recognize and treat all elements of injury or illness in a single emergency department visit.

IF YOUR SYMPTOMS DO NOT IMPROVE OR YOU CANNOT REACH YOUR DOCTOR, YOU MAY RETURN TO THE EMERGENCY DEPARTMENT. MEANWHILE, FOLLOW THE INSTRUCTIONS BELOW AS INDICATED FOR YOU.

Follow-up Procedures – General Instructions

You may return to work: ____ When released by a physician, _____ In _#___ days, or ___ If you are free of symptoms.

An emergency interpretation of X-Rays was provided by the Emergency Physician. A final evaluation will be made by a Radiologist or Internist. You will be contacted if additional treatment is necessary.

Some fractures (broken bones) do not show at the time of original injury, but will show themselves in 10–14 days. Please return for repeat X-Rays if you are not improving.

It is common to find additional bruises and experience greater discomfort the day after an accident. If new injuries are recognized it is important to return for further evaluation.

SUPPLEMENTAL AFTERCARE INSTRUCTIONS

___Croup	__ Animal Bites	__ Ankle Sprain	__ Clear Liquids	__ Hypertension
__ Strep Throat	__ Head injury	__ Fractures	__ Diarrhea	___ Assault Information
__ Upper Respiratory Infections	__ Tetanus Prevention	___ Splints & Casts	__Nausea & Vomiting	__ Other_____
__ Urinary Tract infections	___ Wound care/ suture removal	__ Low Back Pain	__ Eye Injury	_____

INDIVIDUAL INSTRUCTIONS

Increase fluid, increase fiber, and increase exercise. Return if you worsen in any way.

PLEASE RETURN TO THE EMERGENCY ROOM
IF YOU THINK IT IS NECESSARY

I hereby Acknowledge Receipt of my Discharge Instructions and Understand them.

X   _Amy Robertson_____

     Patient

_ _ _ _ _ _ V. Branson, LPN___

Discharge Instructions Given By

Idaho Memorial Hospital
876 Memory Lane, Anywhere, ID 83776
(208) 378-5555

Patient Name	Maiden Name	Date of Birth	Record Number	Date of Admission	Time of Admission
Ramsey, Lyle C.		11/28/xx	410027	11/28/xx	2406

Patient Address	Social Security Number	Gender	Marital Status	Date of Discharge	Time of Discharge
722 Armstead Way Valley View, ID 83752	518-63-9999	M	S	12/03/xx	1900

Patient Telephone Number	Occupation	Birthplace	Religion	Length of Stay	Room Number
208 455-2323		ID	LDS	5	NB

Primary Insurer	Policy and Group Number	Secondary Insurer		Policy Number	Group Number
Blue Shield	56243302	NA		NA	NA

Guarantor Name	Guarantor Relationship	Next of Kin Name			Relationship
Ramsey, Lydia	Mother	Ramsey, Lydia			Mother

Guarantor Address	Guarantor Telephone	Next of Kin Address			Telephone
722 Armstead Way Valley View, ID 83752	208 455-2323	722 Armstead Way Valley View, ID 83752			208 455-2323

Admitting Physician	Service Type	Admit Type	Admitted From	Address	Telephone
Dr. George Barnett	IP	NB	Delivery	722 Armstead Way Valley View, ID 83752	208 455-2323

Attending Physician	Attending Physician UPIN	Admission Diagnosis			
Dr. George Barnett	89526	Full Term New Born via C-Section			

Diagnoses and Procedures

Principle Diagnoses					ICD-9-CM Code
Full-Term Newborn via C-Section					

Secondary Diagnoses					
Jaundiced					

Principle Procedure					
Circumcision					

Secondary Procedure					

Total Charges:	$2489.

179

Idaho Memorial Hospital
876 Memory Lane, Anywhere, ID 83776
(208) 378-5555

Standing Orders for Normal Newborn

Date & Time	Orders	X	Date & Time	Orders
SSnider,RN 2406 11/28/xx	**DELIVERY ROOM** 1. Dry baby well under warmer 2. cover baby including most of head & keep warm. 3. Footprint & place ID bands on both Arms. 4. Aqua Mephyton 1 mg IM		Noted SSnider, RN 11/30/xx 0030	**OBSERVE & REPORT TO DOCTOR ANY OF THE FOLLOWING** 1. Abnormal, absence of, or frequent liquid BMs. 2. Absence of urination or phimosis. 3. Respiratory difficulties; rapid respiration or cyanosis. 4. Jaundice, especially first 24 hours. 5. elevated, low, or unstable temperatures. 6. Persistent feeding problems. 7. Unusual weight loss. 8. Jitteriness.

Noted SSnider, RN 11/29/xx 0030	**ADMISSION ORDER TO NURSERY**
	1. Ilotycin ointment to each eye (ophthalmic ointment)
	2. Weight, length and OFC
	3. Bathe with soap & water, rinse well 4–6 hours after admission or when Temp is 98.6 – NOT BEFORE.
	4. Temperature
	5. Clean cord with alcohol & watch Closely for bleeding & signs of infection.
	6. Keep air passages free of mucus With bulb syringe or deep suction PRN.
	7. Allow mother to hold baby <u>with Nurse in attendance</u> as soon as baby is stabilized.
			12/03/xx 1910 Noted BJenkins, RN	**DAILY ROUTINE CARE**
				1. Daily bath with tap water or baby soap solution. Use no oil on skin.
				2. Temperature each shift.
				3. Feedings: a. NPO 2–6 hours
				   b. D5W feeding x1
				   c. House formula q4hours
				   d. Nursing babies to breast first feeding.
				   e. Supplement nursing babies with D5W only unless House formula requested by mother.
				DISCHARGE ORDERS:
				1. Discharge baby with mother
				2. discharge instructions for Repeat PKU, PRN

x = only the prescribed medication may be dispensed.

Standing Orders for Normal Newborn

Idaho Memorial Hospital
876 Memory Lane, Anywhere, ID 83776
(208) 378-5555

Physician's Orders & Progress Notes

Instructions: Notate progress of case, complications, change in diagnosis, condition on discharge, & instructions to patient.

Date & Time	Orders	X	Date & Time	Progress Notes
11/30/xx	HCT in arm Standing orders/ Dr Barnett			
11/30/xx	Give ¼ cc Hepatitis b vaccine IM With parent consent. S.O. SSnider, RN Dr Barnett			

x = only the prescribed medication may be dispensed.

Physician's Orders & Progress Notes

Idaho Memorial Hospital
876 Memory Lane, Anywhere, ID 83776
(208) 378-5555

Nursing Notes

Date		
12/2	1800	Color is jaundiced. Dr Barnett in to check on baby. Baby appears to be doing well
		.—VS stable.—Alert et responsive to cares. Baby nipples well.—Feedings tolerated
		Well. Infant voids, et BM's. Family & friends handle baby but Mom also does well
		With infant. - - - -Baby has reddened bottom—A&D oint applied
12/3	0530	Baby out w/mom-handled well. Appears to be bonding well.
	0600	- - - - - - - - - - - -HB Domer, RN- -
12/3	0600-	0700 Back to nursery. Alert et active with am cares. Skin warm et pink with sl
	1800	jaundice noted. VS stable Dr Barnett in to check baby. Mom handles baby better.
		Nipples well. Voids et BM's as.- - - - - - - - - - - Sara James, RN
12/3	1800	Color se jaundiced; VS stable Breath sounds clear bil abdomen soft with bowel
	1900	Sounds present. PKU was done; also, HepaVax was given Teaching completed
		Mom verbalized & demonstrates ability to understand teaching & care for infant.- - -
		Circ. Healing, cord dry cont cares taught. Baby is DC to mom in apparently good
		Condition. Mom encouraged to call in case of problems.- - - - - - - - - - -
		DC with Mom in apparently good condition, as also assessed by Dr Barnett.
		- - - - - - - - - - - - - -- - - - - - - - - - - - - -- - - - - - - -HB Domer, RN

Nursing Notes

Idaho Memorial Hospital
876 Memory Lane, Anywhere, ID 83776
(208) 378-5555

Nursing Notes

Date			
	1930	Returned to nursery. Gassy voided & stool, no bleeding circum. Nipples well	
12/1	0100	Nipples well with spitting	
	0500	VS stable. Voiding & stooling qs Out to mother fair bonding- - - -*SaraJames, RN*	
	0730	Back to nursery. Bathed & weighed HOB up @ window—*SJ, RN*	
	1630	SM. Amt yellow puss-like drainage on diaper and on penis & Plastibell. Circ cleaned	
		& Neosporin applied. Out to eat——*SaraJames, RN*	
12/1	1800	Return to nursery by family. Alert & active VS stable. Sl jaundice	
		Alc to dry con & prn. Circ good H&D alert to reddened area on bottom. Fussy DC'd	
		Zit. GS sleeping.	
	2100	-2210 Out with mother. Nippled well & retained feeding	
	2210	Sleeping	
	23-	0230 fussy off & on. Sleeping	
12/2	0500	Out with mother - - - - - - - -*KLevit, LPN*	
		Retained feedings. - - - - - *KLevit, LPN*	
12/2	0600	Alert et active w/AM cares. Skin warm et pink with SL jaundice noted. VS stable.	
	–	Fussy. Talked to Dr. Barnett on baby's status. Out to mom. Mom doing better with	
	1800	feedings. Nipples well. Voids et BM's as. Circ. Ok - - - - *SaraJames, RN*	
	1800	Baby is out with mom. Color pink with SL jaundice – responsive to care. Checked on	
		Often. Family is holding infant. Baby is sleeping. Barnett in to check on infant.	
		- - - - - - - - - - - - - - - -*HB Domer, RN*- - - - - - -	

Nursing Notes

Idaho Memorial Hospital
876 Memory Lane, Anywhere, ID 83776
(208) 378-5555

Nursing Notes

Date		
11/29	0110	Rectal T 98.5 bathed, jittery. One touch 42 nippled without S.ow rare grunt & flare
	0130	Rectal T 98.0 out to mom- - - - - - - - - - - - - - - - - - MBingam, LPN
	0300	Returned to nursery VS stable nippled sips VS good bonding with mom & family
	0500	Sleeping Resp regular- - - - - - - - - - - - - - - - - MBingam, LPN
11/29	0600-	Alert et active with AM cares lab in for HCT VS stable. Skin warm et pink. Dr.
	1800	Barnett in to check baby. Mom handles baby fair to well. Nipples well. Voids as. No
		BM since birth. - - - - - - - - - - - - - - - - - - MBingam, LPN
	1800	Color pink VS stable. Breath sounds clear bil abdomen soft with bowel sounds
		present. Baby voids et BM's SJ- - - - - - - - - - - - - - - - -
11/30	0600	Infant Nipples well - -Feedings tol well - - - - - - - - - - - - - - - - - -
		Appears to be bonding well with mom.- - - - - - - - - - - -HBDomer, RN
11/30	0645	Alert & active during AM cares VS stable pink alcohol to dry cord prn. Nippled
		Ss form sleeping
	0820	Dr Silver in to check for Dr. Barnett. Circ done with 1.2 Plastibell.
	0940	Out with mother good bonding. Baby nippled well with slight spitting
	1030	Back in nursery. ONC good sleeping.
	1300	Out with family. Nippled well. Remains with family
	1430	Back in nursery sleeping
	1600	Mother request baby stay in the nursery – nippled Z sleeping.
	1730	Circ remains good – has voided & BM w/ cs - - - - - - -KLevit, LPN
11/30	1040	Dr John in @ 0900 Hep B vaccine ordered
		1040 Hepatitis B vaccine .25 cc given IM to ® thigh- - -HBDomer, RN

Nursing Notes

Idaho Memorial Hospital

876 Memory Lane, Anywhere, ID 83776
(208) 378-5555

Dear Parent:

In addition to the usual immunizations, there has been a recommendation from the national health authorities to give routine Hepatitis B vaccine to all newborns. This is done by a series of three immunizations – at birth, two months, and six months. The cost for the 1st dose in the hospital is approximately $30.00, which is covered by Medicaid and some insurance companies. The 2nd and 3rd doses can be obtained at the Health Department or at your doctor's office with their usual charges for stated supplies & vaccines.

The incidence of Hepatitis B in Idaho is about one hundred cases per year (= 1/10,000). It can be a serious and sometimes fatal illness. To be protected your child must receive <u>ALL THREE DOSES</u> of the vaccine.

We support the recommendation, but recognize questions exist about cost vs benefit, duration of immunity, and number of shots an infant is receiving. It is expected that routine immunization against Hepatitis B will eventually be standard practice. For now, we believe it should be offered for you to decide at your discretion.

Sincerely ,

Barnett, John, & Blamires

MEDICAL STAFF

I have been offered the Hepatitis B vaccine for my newborn. I have received the printed literature titled "IMPORTANT INFORMATION ABOUT HEPATITIS B, HEPATITIS B VACCINE, AND HEPATITIS B IMMUNE GLOBULIN". By accepting, I agree to follow-up with the second and third doses at 1–2 months and at 6 months.

ACCEPT:

    Date: __11/26/93__

Lydia Ramsey

PARENT'S SIGNATURE

DECLINE:

    Date: _____

PARENT'S SIGNATURE

SSnider, RN

Witness

Newborn Nursing Flowsheet

Idaho Memorial Hospital
876 Memory Lane, Anywhere, ID 83776
(208) 378-5555

Date: 11/28/xx	Hosp Days: 1											2							11/30/xx					
Assessment																								
Time	24	0100	0130	0300	0600	0830	0930	1000	1200	1400	1600	1800	1900	2000	2300	2400	0200	0400	0600	0930	1100	1300	1430	1600
Temp	97^1	97^5	98^2	97^9	98^2	98^4					98^4					98^6			98^2					
Pulse	159	147	148	141	149						146					148			141					
Resp.	39	37	35	36	40						40					40			40					
B/P	81/46																							
Weight	6.1				6.9																			
Time in	x																							
Time out			x	x			x		x	x											x	x	x	
Color	P	P	P	P	P					P		P	P	P	P	P		P	P	P	x	P		
Skin	CM	CM	CM	CM	CM					CM		CM	CM	CM	CM			CM	CM	CM		CM		
Cord Care				x				x	x						x			x	x			x		
Intake																								
Breast																								
Formula				sips		3/1			3/55			3/55		3/1		3/1			3/1	3/85		3/95		3/1
D5W Sterile H2O		.15																						
Comments						T			T			T		T		S			T	S		T		T
Output																								
Urine	x			x					x						x			x				x		
Stool																		x				x		
Emesis																s				s				
Labs																								
Results						51.5																		
Glucose		44																						
Special Instructions																								
Hand & Foot prints																								
Picture																								
Other:																								

Dr. Visit

	gb							gb															
Nurses Initials	MTB	MTB	MTB	MTB	MTB	MTB	MTB	MTB	MTB	MTB	MTB	SJ	SJ	SJ	SJ	SJ	SJ	SJ	HBD	KPL	KPL	KPL	KPL	KPL

Signature Legend

Initials	Signature
Nurses: MTB	MTBingam, LPN
SJ	Sarajanes, RN
HBD	HBDomer, RN
KPL	KLevit, LPN

Physicians:

Initials	Signature
gb	George Barnett, MD
PJ	Phillip John, MD

Charting Legend:

Color	P – Pink	C – Cyanotic	J – Jaundice	D – Dusky
Skin	CM – Clear & Moist	P – Peeling	D – Dry	R – Rash
Intake Comments	E – Encouragement Needed	R – Refused	S – Spitty	T – Tolerated Well
Cord Care	C – Cleaned per Protocol	R – Refused	R – Red	
Activity	JIT – Jittery	IRR – Irritable	L – Lethargic	M – Moves Extremities Well

Newborn Nursing Flowsheet

Date 12/01/xx — Hosp Days: 3

Assessment	1900	0100	0500	0700	1000	1300	1400	1600	1700	1800	2100	2300
Time												
Temp	97^1		98^2		98^2			98^4				
Pulse	137		145		155			175				
Resp.	39		35		40			48				
B/P												
Weight				6.4								
Time in	x		x	x	1040	1100	1310	1430				
Time out									1630			
Color	P	P	P	P	P					P		P
Skin	J	J	J	J	J							
Cord Care	x		x	x					x			
Intake												
Breast												
Formula	3/11	3/11	3/1	3/1	3/11	3/1	3/1			3/11		
D5W Sterile H2O												
Comments												
Output												
Urine	x	x	x		x	xx			x	x	x	x
Stool	i	i	i	i	i	i	i	i	x	x	x	x
Emesis												
Labs												
Results				PKU								
Glucose												
Special Instructions												
Hand & Foot prints												
Picture												
Other:												
Nurses Initials	SAJ	SAJ	SAJ	SAJ	gb / SAJ	SAJ	SAJ	SAJ	KPL	KPL	KPL	KPL

Date 12/02/xx — Hosp Days: 4

Assessment	0100	0500	0600	0800	0900	1100	1300	1400	1600	1800	1900	2200
Time												
Temp	99^3		98^6				99^2					98^5
Pulse	147		135				141					142
Resp.	42		40				41					47
B/P												
Weight				6.5								
Time in		x			x	x			x		x	
Time out												
Color	P	P	P	P		P	P	P		P		
Skin	J	J	J			J	J	J		J	J	J
Cord Care	x		x							x		x
Intake												
Breast												
Formula	3/1		3/1	3/1			3/85			3/95		3/1
D5W Sterile H2O			T	T				T				
Comments												
Output												
Urine	x	x	x	x	x	x	x		x	x	x	x
Stool	x	x	x			x				x		x
Emesis												
Labs												
Results												
Glucose												
Nurses Initials	KPL	KPL	KPL	KPL	KPL	KPL	KPL	KPL	KPL	HBD	SAJ	SAJ

Dr. Visit / Signature Legend

Nurses Initials	Signature
MTB	Bingam, LPN
SAJ	Sarajames, RN
KPL	KLevit, LPN
HBD	HBDomer, RN

Physicians: gb — George Barnett, MD

Charting Legend:

Color	Skin	Intake Comments	Cord Care	Activity
P-Pink	CM – Clear & Moist	E – Encouragement Needed	C – Cleaned per Protocol	JIT – Jittery
C-Cyanotic	P – Peeling	R – Refused	R – Red	IRR – Irritable
J-Jaundice	D – Dry	S – Spitty		L – Lethargic
D- Dusky	R – Rash	T – Tolerated Well		M – Moves Extremities Well

Newborn Nursing Flowsheet

Idaho Memorial Hospital
876 Memory Lane, Anywhere, ID 83776
(208) 378-5555

Date: 12/03/xx	Hosp Days: 5											
Assessment	2400	0200	0400	0500	0700	0900	1100	1300	1400	1600	1700	1800
Temp	99^1				98^2			99^2			98^4	
Pulse	131				140			139			146	
Resp.	45				40			42			44	
B/P												
Weight					6.6							
Time in						x	x	x	x	x		
Time out												
Color	J		J	J	J	J	J	J	J		J	J
Skin	CM			CM	CM			CM		CM	CM	CM
Cord Care	x			x				x			x	x
Intake												
Breast												
Formula				sips		3/1			3/55		3/55	3/55
D5W Sterile H2O		.15										
Comments				T		T			T		T	T
Output												
Urine	x	x	x	x	x	x	x	x	x	x	x	x
Stool	x	x	x	x	x	x	x	x	x	x	x	x
Emesis												
Labs												
Results												
Glucose												
Special Instructions												
Hand & Foot prints												
Picture												
Other:												

Dr. Visit												
Nurses Initials	HBD	HBD	HBD	HBD	SAJ	gb SAJ	SAJ	SAJ	SAJ	SAJ	SAJ	SAJ

Signature Legend	Initials	Signature		Initials	Signature		Initials	Signature		Initials	Signature
Nurses:	HBD	HB Dower, RN									
	SAJ	Sara James, RN									
	KPL	K Levit, LPN									

Physicians:	gb	George Barnett, MD

Charting Legend:

Color	P-Pink	C-Cyanotic	J-Jaundice	D- Dusky
Skin	CM – Clear & Moist	P – Peeling	D – Dry	R – Rash
Intake Comments	E – Encouragement Needed	R – Refused	S – Spitty	T – Tolerated Well
Cord Care	C – Cleaned per Protocol		R – Red	
Activity	JIT – Jittery	IRR – Irritable	L – Lethargic	M – Moves Extremities Well

Idaho Memorial Hospital
876 Memory Lane, Anywhere, ID 83776
(208) 378-5555

Patient Name	Maiden Name	Date of Birth	Record Number	Date of Admission	Time of Admission
Thomas, Garrett		01/22/xx	410028	02/22/xx	0910

	Social Security Number	Gender			Date of Discharge	Time of Discharge
Patient Address	412505378	M			02/22/xx	1410
Rt 4 Box 520 Valley View, ID 83752						

Patient Telephone Number	Occupation		Birthplace	Religion	Length of Stay	Room Number
208-532-4438	High School Student		ID	Prot	1	OPS

Primary Insurer	Policy and Group Number		Secondary Insurer		Policy Number	Group Number
Blue Shield	412505378		NA		NA	NA

Guarantor Name	Guarantor Relationship		Next of Kin Name			Relationship
Richards, Mary E.	Mother		Richards, Patrick			Father

Guarantor Address	Guarantor Telephone		Next of Kin Address			Telephone
647 Armstead Way Valley View, ID 83752	208 455-3245		647 Armstead Way Valley View, ID 83752			208 455-3245

Admitting Physician	Service Type		Admit Type	Admitted From	Address	Telephone
Dr. Floyd West	OPS		OPS	Home	647 Armstead Way Valley View, ID 83752	208 455-3245

Attending Physician	Attending Physician UPIN		Admission Diagnosis			
Dr. Floyd West	67578		Open Wound Left Tibia			

Diagnoses and Procedures						ICD-9-CM Code
Principle Diagnoses						
Subacute and chronic colitis						
Secondary Diagnoses						
Grade 2 adenocarcinoma						
Principle Procedure						
Colonoscopy						
Secondary Procedure						

Total Charges:	$2489.					

Idaho Memorial Hospital
876 Memory Lane, Anywhere, ID 83776
(208) 378-5555

OUTPATIENT SURGERY

LAST NAME	FIRST NAME	MIDDLE	AGE	BIRTHDATE	PHONE	DATE
Thomas	Garrett		44	01/22/xx	208–532-4438	2/22/xx

RESPONSIBLE PARTY NAME	RESP. PARTY ADDRESS	CITY/STATE/ZIP	EMPLOYER
____Same____	Rt 4 Box 520 ___	Valley View, ID 83752	Self__ ___

INSURANCE CO. NO.	GROUP INS. WITH	POLICY NO.	POLICY HOLDER
____Blue Cross of Id_____ __		412505378_____	_____ _

TIME	BP	TPR	NURSING REMARKS
0910	122/78	96.7 84-16	OPS- colonoscopy. Preop teaching done. 22 gauge 5 1/2 NS 1000 cc TKO ® hand per Dr. West.— DKood, RN
1220			Return from endoscopy per cart w/rails up. sleeping
1330	134/80	84-16	Dr. With pt. May discharge when pt ready. Up to bathroom.
			Tolerate activity. IV DC'd 400 cc infused
1410			Wanted to leave. Up and dressed.

LIST ANY ALLERGIES OR OTHER SPECIAL INFORMATION	NURSE'S SIGNATURE	PATIENT CONDITION ON DISCHARGE:
none	DKood, RN	Good/tol activity

PHYSICIAN'S REPORT	States understands diet. Home with Dad to drive. – DKood, RN
- -West	

DIAGNOSIS:

TREATMENT:

DISPOSITION:

AUTHORIZATION FOR MEDICAL and/or SUGICAL TREATMENT:

x_____

I hereby authorize Dr. _____to administer   SIGNATURE OF PATIENT
Such treatment as is, in his judgment, necessary:

INSTRUCTIONS TO PATIENT:	

PATIENT SIGNATURE   DATE   TIME   PHYSICIAN SIGNATURE

Idaho Memorial Hospital
876 Memory Ln, Anywhere, ID 83776
(208) 378-5555

Colonoscopy Report

Date of Procedure: 2-22-xx

INDICATIONS: 44-year-old male with an approximately 24-month history of diarrhea. He has taken Azulfidine inter-mittently and apparently with good results. He also has a brother with ulcerative colitis. He describes multiple barium enemas over time as being normal. One a couple of years ago in Rupert raises the question of ulcerative colitis with loss of haustration in the left colon and possible mucosal involvement. He rarely sees blood in his stool, however, recently he had a flu-like syndrome with recurrent diarrhea. On this occasion it has not responded to Azulfidine even with an increase from 4 tablets to 8 tablets a day. He has never been colonoscoped. Due to long-standing history of possible ulcerative colitis as well as refractory symptoms and some uncertainty about the basic diagnosis, total colonoscopy is planned. He has undergone a Co-Lyte prep consisting of two liters of Co-Lyte since he is having 8–9 stools per day.

EXAMINATION: Following informed consent, he was sedated with Demerol 50 mg, Phenergan 25 mg, and Versed 1 mg IV. During the exam he was given an additional 25 mg of Demerol. The scope was introduced and advanced to what was thought to be cecum. The cecal tip could not be seen but there was marked deformity and what was felt to be ileocecal valve was easily visualized. It could not be entered despite repeated attempts. A picture was taken. Fluid could be seen refluxing from the apparent valve. There was a small area of ulceration near this and this was included in the previously noted picture. The scope was withdrawn with detailed inspection of the mucosa. There were also scattered ulcers with moderate depth. These were associated with some friability. The colitis had a segmental distrib-ution with apparently normal intervening mucosa. At 30 cm. On withdrawal a polyp also seen on introduction of the scope was seen and pictures taken. It is semi-circumferential. There is some friability. The overall size of the polyp is estimated at 3 cm. and it is very sessile. Multiple biopsies were taken. Two pictures were also taken. Scattered biop-sies were taken from throughout the colon and submitted as colon and rectum. There was also an area of serpigi-nous ulceration in the rectum. I should note that there was no active inflammation at the level of the sigmoid polyp. Anal was unremarkable and no fissures or fistulae were seen. He tolerated the procedure well.

FINAL IMPRESSION:
1. The colonic appearance is most suggestive of Crohn's disease. Unfortunately, terminal ileum could not be visualized.
2. Large sigmoid polyp – suspicious based on appearance for malignancy.

PLAN: He will continue Azulfidine for now and will be notified with the biopsy reports. A report will also be sent to Dr. Shirley, his primary care physician in Valley View. He will require surgical resection of the sigmoid polyp and will probably require corticosteroid therapy.

F. West, MD

Floyd West, MD

FW: shc
2-22-xx/2-25-xx
#1
cc: office
Dr. C. Shirley, Valley View

Idaho Memorial Hospital
876 Memory Lane, Anywhere, ID 83776
(208) 378-5555

Endoscopy Record
Physical Assessment Data

Date: 02/22/xx Procedure Start Time: 1125			Procedure End Time: 1220				
Allergies: none							

Procedure:		**# Specimen to lab**	Time	O$_2$ SAT	BP	PULSE	INIT.
	Bronchoscopy		1125	89	120/79	72	DPW
x	Colonoscopy		1140	89	122/90	80	DPW
	Dilation		1150	93	137/88	70	DPW
	EGD		1200	91	125/91	82	DPW
	ERCP		1210	92	124/87	73	DPW
	Flex Sigmoidoscopy		1215	90	120/85	70	DPW
	Motility						
	Bile Study						
x	Biopsy	3					
	Brushing						
	Polypectomy						
	Washing						
	Other:						
	Other:						

Safety:		**Indicate Location on patient:**	**Medications:**				
	EKG		Drug	Dose	Method	Time	By Whom
	VS Monitor		Demerol	50 mgml	IVP	1120	DKood RN
	Grounding Pad (Lot #)		Phenergan	25 mgml	IVP	1153	DKood RN
	Safety Strap		Versed	1 mgml	IVP	1131	DKood RN
	IV		Demerol	25 mgml	IVP	1155	DKood RN
	Cautery Unit (ID#)						
	Scope (#)						
x	Pulse Oximeter	Left forefinger	IV:			DC @	
x	Side Rails Up	na	O$_2$ L/min	Start:	Mask Cannula	DC @	

Endoscopy Record Physical Assessment Data pg 1

Patient Assessment: Final assessment score must be 12–14 or approved by physician. Any score <2 requires comment in notes column. Patients may not be discharged with any one score of "0" without documented physician notification.

	Pre-Procedure	Assessment score and criteria	Post-Procedure	Notes:
IV Site Check	1125	Patient free from redness and swelling	1220	
Teaching	x	Pre-Procedure instructions given Post-Procedure instructions given	x	
Respiratory	2	2. Respirations adequate Deep breaths – coughs, adequate rate, rhythm & depth. 1. Limited or shallow breaths. 0. Apnea	2	

Circulatory	2	2. B/P stabilized and within patient's normal limits ±20.
		   Pulse-rate, rhythm, quality w/n normal limits ±20.
		1. Blood pressure fluctuating ±30 of baseline pressure.
		   Pulse-rate, rhythm, quality w/n normal limits ±30.
		0. B/P fluctuating ±50 of baseline, B/P <75/40. Pulse-thready, weak
			2	

Color	2	2. Normal Skin color and condition. 1. Change in skin color and/or condition. Color is pale, jaundiced, dusky, or flushed. 0. Frank cyanosis of skin, bluish, gray or purple.	2	
Level of Consciousness	2	2. Alert and oriented (patient is aware of surroundings & what has taken place). 1. Arouses to name, responds to verbal stimuli. 0. Unconscious or difficult to arouse.	2	
Ability to Ambulate	2	2. Able to move/ambulate consistent with pre-admission assessment. 1. Able to move/ambulate only with assistance. 0. Unable to move/ambulate.	2	
Pain	2	2. Complains of no pain or mild pain, relieved by medication. 1. Definite pain causing obvious discomfort, unrelieved by medication. 0. Severe pain, unrelieved by medication.	2	
Nausea & Vomiting	2	2. Absence of nausea. 1. Some nausea/occasional vomiting, tolerates sips of fluid. 0. Uncontrolled nausea and vomiting that prohibits the patient from attempting to retain any oral fluids	2	
Total	14		14	

Disposition – Transfer To:		Discharge Time:		Nurses Notes: skin color pale- Post-op diagnosis: Ulcerative colitis/Crohn's disease DKoodRN
VIA:	W/C		Home With:	
	Ambulatory			
	Stretcher	x	Relationship:	
	Pt. Room OPS	x		MD: Signature/Init: F. West, MD Assistant/Title/Init: M. Watson, STA

Endoscopy Record Physical Assessment Data pg 2

Canyon Pathology Associates
873 NW 15th Ave.
Anywhere, ID 83776

PATHOLOGY REPORT

PATIENT: __Thomas, Garrett__   AGE: __44__

ACC. NO: __CPA-91-554__   HOS. NO: __410028__   DATE: __02/22/xx__

SNOP NO: DOCTOR: __West__

OPERATION: COLONOSCOPY
                 #1 CECUM
                 #2 30 CM.
                 #3 RECTAL
                 ULCERATIVE COLITIS?, CROHN'S DISEASE

GROSS: Specimen #1 consists of several, pink-tan tissues that are up to 0.6 cm. in largest dimension. They are processed as received. Specimen #2 consists of multiple, similar, pink-tan tissues that are also up to 0.6 cm. in largest dimension. They are processed as received. Specimen #3 is a similar, pink-tan tissue up to 0.6 cm. It is also processes as received. EEF/sg/2-25-91

MICRO: Specimen #1 reveals fragments of colonic mucosa throughout which is both an acute and chronic inflammatory exudate. Numerous eosinophils are also present. Muscularis mucosae is present within some fragments. There is some mucosal flattening. No discrete ulceration is present, nor are there discrete crypt abscesses present. Where submucosa is present, no granulomata are seen. There is minimal inflammation present below the muscularis mucosae. Specimen #2 from the 30 cm. position of the colon reveals severe dysplasia with decreased mucin production, pseudostratification of the nuclei, and increased mitotic activity. The changes present are consistent with a Grade 2 adenocarcinoma. Specimen #3 reveals findings similar to those described in Specimen #1.

NOTE: The changes seen in both Specimens #1 and #3 would be consistent with CUC. They do not, however, completely exclude Crohn's disease.

Specimen #1, subacute and chronic colitis, severe, non-specific.
Specimen #2, Grade 2 adenocarcinoma.
Specimen #3, subacute and chronic colitis, severe, non-specific.
                                         (SEE NOTE)

Thomas, Garrett 05-43-69

                                        Christopher Omart, MD

                                         Christopher Omart, M.D. PATHOLOGIST

PATHOLOGY REPORT

Idaho Memorial Hospital
876 Memory Ln, Anywhere, ID 83776
(208) 378-5555

CONSENT TO OPERATION

PATIENT: _____Garrett Thomas_____   __Age: 44 yrs_____

Date: __2-22-xx__   Time: __0920 am__   Place: Idaho Memorial Hospital

1. I hereby authorize Dr. West_____ and whomever he may designate as his/her assistants, to perform upon __myself_____. The following operations: __Colonoscopy w/poss biopsy, poss polypectomy__ and in any unforeseen conditions arises in the course of the operation, calling in his judgment for procedures in addition to, or different from, those now contemplated, I further request and authorize him to do whatever he deems advisable.

2. The nature and purpose of the operation, possible alternative methods of treatment, the risks involved, and the possibility of complications have been explained to me. I acknowledge that no guarantee or assurance has been made the results that may be obtained.

3. I consent to the administration of anesthesia, and to the use of such anesthetics as the attending physician, anesthesiologist, and the hospital staff may deem advisable. I understand that all anesthetics involve risks or complications, serious injury, or rarely, death from both known and unknown causes, and that no guarantees have been made as to the results of the anesthetic.

4. I consent to the disposal, by authorities of Idaho Memorial Hospital, of any tissues or parts which may have been removed.

5. For the purpose of advancing medical and nursing education, I consent to the admittance of the personnel to the operating room.

I CERTIFY THAT I HAVE READ AND FULLY UNDERSTAND THE ABOVE CONSENT TO OPERATION, THAT THE EXPLANATIONS THEREIN REFERRED TO WERE MADE AND THAT ALL BLANKS FOR COMLETION WERE FILLED IN AND INAPPLICABLE PARAGRAPHS, IF ANY, WERE STRICKEN BEFORE I SIGNED.

GTHOMAS

_____
SIGNATURE OF PATIENT

_____
SIGNATURE OF PATIENT'S HUSBAND OR WIFE

When patient is a minor or incompetent to give consent:

_____
SIGNATURE OF PERSON AUTHORIZED TO CONSENT TO PATIENT

_____
RELATIONSHIP TO PATIENT

D.Kood, RN

_____
WITNESS

Idaho Memorial Hospital
876 Memory Lane, Anywhere, ID 83776
(208) 378-5555

Physician's Orders & Progress Notes

Instructions: Notate progress of case, complications, change in diagnosis, condition on discharge, & instructions to patient.

Date & Time	Orders	X	Date & Time	Progress Notes
			2/22/91	DIAGNOSIS: ?UC x 24 yrs PLANNED PROCEDURE: colonoscopy INFORMED CONSENT: yes PREOPERATIVE REVIEW OF BODY SYSTEMS: CARDIOVASCULAR: 0 PULMONARY: 0 OTHER: 0 REGULAR MEDICATIONS: Azulfidine ALLERGIES: NKA BLEEDING/CLOTTING DISORDERS: 0 DETAILED H&P DICTATED: 0 SIGNATURE: __F. West, MD__

x = only the prescribed medication may be dispensed.

Physician's Orders   Progress Notes

Idaho Memorial Hospital
876 Memory Lane, Anywhere, ID 83776
(208) 378-5555

OUTPATIENT – LOCAL PRE-OPERATIVE CHECKLIST

NAME: Garrett Thomas   Dr. West   DATE: 02-22-xx

SURGICAL PROCEDURE: Colonoscopy

V/S: T   96.7   P   84   R   16   BP   122/78   H

WT: 195 lbs   AGE: 44

ALLERGIES: none

What routine medications does the patient currently take?   Azulfidine.

Does the patient have any pre-existing health problems: (i.e. heart, lungs)   No.

Does the patient have a pacemaker: NO   Is the patient diabetic?   No

Has the patient ever had hepatitis?   yes   WHEN: 1976

Level of awareness: Understands surgery? X   Oriented to person?   X   Place?   X

Time?   X

Level of anxiety: Minimal   X   Moderate: Severe

Fears, Misconceptions: none

SURGICAL CHECK LIST

Is the surgical permit signed?   X

Does it agree with the surgery scheduled?   X

Is the ID band on the Right wrist   X

When did the patient last eat or drink?   Cranberry juice this am

HAVE THE FOLLOWING BEEN REMOVED?

Hearing Aids, earrings   X

Dentures, dental bridges, partial plates   X

Contact Lenses   X   Glasses X

Kari Varigated, RN
_____
Signature of Nurse

Idaho Memorial Hospital
876 Memory Lane, Anywhere, ID 83776
(208) 378-5555

Outpatient Surgery Discharge Instructions

FOR PATIENTS WHO HAVE HAD GENERAL ANESTHESIA, REGIONAL ANESTHESIA OR ANY TYPE OF SEDATION:

1. For the rest of today, the patient may look as if he/she has a slight fever; face might be red, and skin might feel warm and sweaty. The medication given before surgery usually causes this to happen.

2. The medicine which was used to put the patient to sleep will be acting in the patient's body for the next twenty-four (24) hours, so the patient might feel a little sleepy; this feeling will slowly wear off. Because the medicine is still in the patient's system, for the next twenty-four hours the adult patient should not:
   A. drive a car, operate machinery, or power tools,
   B. drink any alcoholic drinks (not even beer), or
   C. make any important decision, such as sign important papers.

3. The patient may have some pain. A prescription for pain may be given by the doctor. This should be taken as directed; and if it does not decrease the pain, contact the patient's doctor. If the doctor does not prescribe anything for pain, the patient may take a non-prescription, non-aspirin pain medication which can be purchased at the drugstore. Please follow the directions on the label.

4. The patient may eat anything, but it is better to start with liquids; such as, water or juice, then soup and crackers, and gradually work up to solid foods. Babies may be fed their milk as soon as they are hungry.

5. The patient is not expected to have any fever; but if the patient does feel warm after today, take his/her temperature. If the temperature is 101 degrees, or higher call the patient's doctor.

6. We strongly suggest that a responsible adult be with the patient for the rest of the day and also during the night for the patient's protection and safety.

7. If any questions arise, call the patient's doctor. If unable to reach the patient's doctor, please feel free to call out-patient surgery. During the day (5 am-5 pm) Monday through Friday, you may call 208-322-7575. At night or on weekends, call the Emergency Department at 208-322-7570.

D.Kood, RN	2-22-xx	9:20am		GThomas	2/22/xx	9:20am
Nurse Signature	Date	Time		Patient Signature	Date	Time

8. The patient has an appointment with Dr. _____

   Date: _____ Time: _____

9. Call Doctor _____ to make an appointment.

Special Instructions: **If you haven't heard from Dr. West by Tuesday afternoon, call his office for report on biopsy 235-2242.

D.Kood, RN	2-22-xx	1410		GThomas	2/22/xx	1410
Nurse Signature	Date	Time		Patient Signature	Date	Time

Outpatient Surgery Discharge Instructions

Idaho Memorial Hospital
876 Memory Lane, Anywhere, ID 83776
(208) 378-5555

Patient Name	Maiden Name		Date of Birth	Record Number	Date of Admission	Time of Admission
Hall , Shelly	Church		05/22/xx	410030	08/26/xx	0930
Patient Address	**Social Security Number**	**Gender**	**Race**	**Marital Status**	**Date of Discharge**	**Time of Discharge**
26469 E. AMITY Way KENORA, ID 83756	577-56-3322	F	C	S	08/26/xx	1105
Patient Telephone Number	**Occupation**		**Birthplace**	**Religion**	**Length of Stay**	**Room Number**
208 658-3359	CLERK-WALMART		ID	Prot	1	OPS
Primary Insurer	**Policy and Group Number**		**Secondary Insurer**		**Policy Number**	**Group Number**
Blue Cross of OR	478815958		NA		NA	NA
Guarantor Name	**Guarantor Relationship**		**Next of Kin Name**			**Relationship**
Self	self		Hall, Patrick			brother
Guarantor Address	**Guarantor Telephone**		**Next of Kin Address**			**Telephone**
26469 E. Amity Way Kenora, ID 83756	208 658-3359		26469 E. Amity Way Kenora, ID 83756			208 658-3359
Admitting Physician	**Service Type**		**Admit Type**	**Admitted From**	**Address**	**Telephone**
Dr. Jeremy Patheal	OPS		OPS	Home	26469 E. Amity Way Kenora, ID 83756	208 658-3359
Attending Physician	**Attending Physician UPIN**		**Admission Diagnosis**			
Dr. Jeremy Patheal	69524		Dysphagia for solids			
Diagnoses and Procedures						
Principle Diagnoses						**ICD-9-CM Code**
Schatzki's Ring						
Secondary Diagnoses						
Dysphagia						
Principle Procedure						
EGD & dilation.						
Secondary Procedure						
Total Charges:	$3589.					

Idaho Memorial Hospital
876 Memory Ln, Anywhere, ID 83776
(208) 378-5555

OUTPATIENT SURGERY

LAST NAME	FIRST NAME	MIDDLE	AGE	BIRTHDATE	PHONE	DATE
Hall	Shelly		55	5/22/xx	208-658-3359	08/26/xx

RESPONSIBLE PARTY NAME	RESP.PARTY ADDRESS	CITY/STATE/ZIP	EMPLOYER
Same			Wal Mart

INSURANCE CO.	NO.	GROUP INS. WITH	POLICY NO	POLICY HOLDER
Blue Cross of OR	478815958	Blue Cross of OR		

TIME	BP	TPR	NURSING REMARKS
0930	160/96	84-16	OPS – Gastroscopy with poss. Bx, Poss Esophageal
			Dilatioin. Preop teaching done. 22 Ga. NS lock ® hand
			Per Dr. Davis
1030			Return from endoscopy. Nauseated.
1105			25 mg Phenergan 12 cc IVP for nausea per Dr. Crane
			May discharge when ready

LIST ANY ALLERGIES OR OTHER SPECIAL INFORMATION	NURSE'S SIGNATURE	PATIENT CONDITION ON DISCHARGE:
Codeine	LBaker, RN	Good/1200-038 150/78

PHYSICIAN'S REPORT	72-16. NS lock Dc'd States feels a little better. Dressed.
-- Patheal	

DIAGNOSIS:

States understands inst. Home with another person to drive --- JPatheal

TREATMENT:

DISPOSITION:

AUTHORIZATION FOR MEDICAL and/or SUGICAL TREATMENT:

x_____

I hereby authorize Dr. _____ to administer   SIGNATURE OF PATIENT
Such treatment as is, in his judgment, necessary:

INSTRUCTIONS TO PATIENT:	

_____x_____x_____

PATIENT SIGNATURE   DATE/TIME   PHYSICIAN SIGNATURE   DATE/TIME

Idaho Memorial Hospital
876 Memory Ln, Anywhere, ID 83776
(208) 378-5555

CONSENT TO OPERATION

PATIENT: ___Shelly Hall_____ Age: 55 yrs _____

Date: ___8-26-xx___ Time: _0935 am_____ Place: Idaho Memorial Hospital

1. I hereby authorize Dr. Patheal_____ and whomever he may designate as his/her assistants, to perform upon __myself_____. The following operations:__Esophagogastroduodenoscopy &/or dilation/poss biopsy___ and in any unforeseen conditions arises in the course of the operation, calling in his judgment for procedures in addition to, or different from, those now contemplated, I further request and authorize him to do whatever he deems advisable.
2. The nature and purpose of the operation, possible alternative methods of treatment, the risks involved, and the possibility of complications have been explained to me. I acknowledge that no guarantee or assurance has been made the results that may be obtained.
3. I consent to the administration of anesthesia, and to the use of such anesthetics as the attending physician, anesthesiologist, and the hospital staff may deem advisable. I understand that all anesthetics involve risks or complications, serious injury, or rarely, death from both known and unknown causes, and that no guarantees have been made as to the results of the anesthetic.
4. I consent to the disposal, by authorities of Idaho Memorial Hospital, of any tissues or parts which may have been removed.
5. For the purpose of advancing medical and nursing education, I consent to the admittance of the personnel to the operating room.

I CERTIFY THAT I HAVE READ AND FULLY UNDERSTAND THE ABOVE CONSENT TO OPERATION, THAT THE EXPLANATIONS THEREIN REFERRED TO WERE MADE AND THAT ALL BLANKS FOR COMLETION WERE FILLED IN AND INAPPLICABLE PARAGRAPHS, IF ANY, WERE STRICKEN BEFORE I SIGNED.

Shelly Hall
_____
SIGNATURE OF PATIENT

_____
SIGNATURE OF PATIENT'S HUSBAND OR WIFE

When patient is a minor or incompetent to give consent:

_____
SIGNATURE OF PERSON AUTHORIZED TO CONSENT TO PATIENT

_____
RELATIONSHIP TO PATIENT

LBaker, RN
_____
WITNESS

ESOPHAGOGASTRODUODENOSCOPY& ESOPHAGEAL DILATATION REPORT

DATE OF OPERATION: 08/26/xx

INDICATIONS: 55-year-old female with a long history of intermittent dysphagia to solids. She has had meat bolus impactions that have lasted several hours at times. She has only rare reflux symptoms but these are not striking. She is a non smoker and there has been no associated weight loss. The dysphagia is somewhat unpredictable.

EXAMINATION: Following informed consent she was sedated with Demerol 50 mg and Versed 1½ mg IV. An Olympus OES type GIF-XQ10 endoscope was introduced. There was a ring of the distal esophagus best seen on retroflex exam of the cardia. There was no endoscopic esophagitis. The remainder of the stomach is unrevealing as is pylorus, duodenal bulb, and several centimeters of post-bulbar duodenum. The endoscope was removed and she was dilated with Maloney type dilators beginning at 46 French and advancing to 50 and 52 French. There was a small amount of blood on the 50 French dilator. She tolerated the procedure well and there were no complications acutely. Following the procedure she did develop some nausea and was given some intravenous Phenergan.

PLAN: Home when ambulatory. May resume regular diet today. She will notify me for any questions or complications.

JPatheal
_____
Jeremy Patheal, M.D.

JP: jbp
08/26/xx-08/27/xx

CC: office

Idaho Memorial Hospital
876 Memory Lane, Anywhere, ID 83776
(208) 378-5555

Date: 11-26-91

PROCEDURE REPORT: DICTATED __X___

INDICATIONS FOR PROCEDURE: _____

PRE-PROCEDURE DIAGNOSTIC STUDIES: _____

PROCEDURE: __Demerol IV Versed 1.5 mg IV_____

FINDINGS & TECHNIQUES: ___ECD – Schatzki's ring with dilation employed without complications & revision Maloney dilators with 46, 50 & 52 F dilation with small amt of blood. _____

PATIENT CONDITION: _____

POST DISCHARGE INSTRUCTIONS: __home when ambulatory _____

DISCHARGE DIAGNOSIS: Schatzki's ring & dilated _____

PHYSICIAN'S SIGNATURE: JPatheal, MD _____

Idaho Memorial Hospital
876 Memory Lane, Anywhere, ID 83776
(208) 378-5555

Endoscopy Record
Physical Assessment Data

Date: 08/26/xx	Procedure Start Time: 1005		Procedure End Time: 1030				
Allergies: codeine							

	Procedure:	# Specimen to lab	Time	O2 SAT	BP	PULSE	INIT.
	Bronchoscopy		1005	94	145/82	65	LBaker, RN
	Colonoscopy		1010	92	163/103	73	LBaker, RN
x	Dilation		1015	93	175/108	72	LBaker, RN
x	EGD		1025	90	173/82	71	LBaker, RN
	ERCP		1030	91	177/84	72	LBaker, RN
	Flex Sigmoidoscopy		1033	88	165/101	69	LBaker, RN
	Motility						
	Bile Study						
	Biopsy	3					
	Brushing						
	Polypectomy						
	Washing						
	Other:						
	Other:						

	Safety:	Indicate Location on patient:	Medications:				
	EKG		Drug	Dose	Method	Time	By Whom
	VS Monitor		Demerol	50 mgml	IVP	1005	LBaker, RN
	Grounding Pad (Lot #)		Versed	1.5 mgml	IVP	1020	LBaker, RN
	Safety Strap		NS	2 cc			
	IV						
	Cautery Unit (ID#)						
x	Scope (# CF × Q10)						
x	Pulse Oximeter	Left forefinger	V:.			DC @	
x	Side Rails Up	na	O2 L/min	Start:	Mask Cannula	DC @	

Endoscopy Record Physical Assessment Data pg 1

Patient Assessment: Final assessment score must be 12–14 or approved by physician. Any score <2 requires comment in notes column. Patients may not be discharged with any one score of "0" without documented physician notification.

	Pre-Procedure	Assessment score and criteria	Post-Procedure	Notes:
IV Site Check	1005	Patient free from redness and swelling	1033	
Teaching	x	Pre-Procedure instructions given Post-Procedure instructions given	x	

Respiratory	2	2. Respirations adequate
		    Deep breaths – coughs, adequate rate, rhythm
		    & depth.
		1. Limited or shallow breaths.
		0. Apnea
			2	

Circulatory	2	2. B/P stabilized and within patient's normal limits ±20.
		    Pulse-rate, rhythm, quality w/n normal limits ±20.
		1. Blood pressure fluctuating ±30 of baseline pressure.
		    Pulse-rate, rhythm, quality w/n normal limits ±30.
		0. B/P fluctuating ±50 of baseline, B/P <75/40. Pulse-thready, weak
			2	

Color	2	2. Normal Skin color and condition. 1. Change in skin color and/or condition. Color is pale, jaundiced, dusky, or flushed. 0. Frank cyanosis of skin, bluish, gray or purple.	2	
Level of Consciousness	2	2. Alert and oriented (patient is aware of surroundings & what has taken place). 1. Arouses to name, responds to verbal stimuli. 0. Unconscious or difficult to arouse.	2	
Ability to Ambulate	2	2. Able to move/ambulate consistent with pre-admission assessment. 1. Able to move/ambulate only with assistance. 0. Unable to move/ambulate.	2	

Pain	2	2. Complains of no pain or mild pain, relieved by
		    medication.
		1. Definite pain causing obvious discomfort, unrelieved
		    by medication.
		0. Severe pain, unrelieved by medication.
			2	

Nausea & Vomiting	2	2. Absence of nausea.
		1. Some nausea/occasional vomiting, tolerates sips
		    of fluid.
		0. Uncontrolled nausea and vomiting that prohibits the
		    patient from attempting to retain any oral fluids
			2	

Total	14		14	

Disposition – Transfer To:			Discharge Time:1035	Nurses Notes: skin color pale- Post-op diagnosis: Schatzki's Ring – Dilated
VIA:	W/C		Home With:	
	Ambulatory			
	Stretcher	x	Relationship:	JPatheal, MD LBaker, RN
	Pt. Room OPS	x		MD: Signature/Init: Assistant/Title/Init:

Endoscopy Record Physical Assessment Data pg 2

(continued)

Idaho Memorial Hospital
876 Memory Lane, Anywhere, ID 83776
(208) 3785555

Physician's Orders & Progress Notes

Instructions: Notate progress of case, complications, change in diagnosis, condition on discharge, & instructions to patient.

Date & Time	Orders	X	Date & Time	Progress Notes
			08/26/xx	DIAGNOSIS: Dysphagia for solids PLANNED PROCEDURE: EGD & poss dilation INFORMED CONSENT: yes PREOPERATIVE REVIEW OF BODY SYSTEMS: CARDIOVASCULAR: 0 high HTN PULMONARY: 0 OTHER: REGULAR MEDICATIONS: Hidiuril, Hytrin ALLERGIES: Codeine BLEEDING/CLOTTING DISORDERS: 0 DETAILED H&P DICTATED: 0 SIGNATURE: JPatheal, MD

x = only the prescribed medication may be dispensed.

Physician's Orders   Progress Notes

Idaho Memorial Hospital
876 Memory Lane, Anywhere, ID 83776
(208) 378-5555

OUTPATIENT – LOCAL PRE-OPERATIVE CHECKLIST

NAME: <u>Shelly Hall</u>   Dr. <u>Patheal</u>   DATE: <u>11-26-91</u>

SURGICAL PROCEDURE: <u>EGD with dilation</u>

WT: <u>220 lbs</u>   AGE: <u>55</u>

ALLERGIES: <u>Codeine</u>

What routine medications does the patient currently take? <u>Hidiuril; Hytrin.</u>

Does the patient have any pre-existing health problems: (i.e. heart, lungs) <u>high BP.</u>

Does the patient have a pacemaker: <u>No</u>   Is the patient diabetic? <u>No</u>

Has the patient ever had hepatitis? <u>No</u>

Level of awareness: Understands surgery? <u>X</u>   Oriented to person? <u>X</u>   Place? <u>X</u>

Time? <u>X</u>

Level of anxiety: Minimal <u>X</u>   Moderate: _____   Severe _____

Fears, Misconceptions: <u>none</u>

<u>SURGICAL CHECK LIST</u>

Is the surgical permit signed? <u>X</u>

Does it agree with the surgery scheduled? <u>X</u>

Is the ID band on the Right wrist <u>X</u>

When did the patient last eat or drink? <u>Before MN</u>

HAVE THE FOLLOWING BEEN REMOVED?

Hearing Aids, earrings <u>X</u>

Dentures, dental bridges, partial plates <u>X</u>

Contact Lenses <u>X</u>   Glasses <u>X</u>

LBaker, RN
_____
Signature of Nurse

Idaho Memorial Hospital
876 Memory Lane, Anywhere, ID 83776
(208) 378-5555

Outpatient Surgery Discharge Instructions

FOR PATIENTS WHO HAVE HAD GENERAL ANESTHESIA, REGIONAL ANESTHESIA OR ANY TYPE OF SEDATION:

1. For the rest of today, the patient may look as if he/she has a slight fever; face might be red, and skin might feel warm and sweaty. The medication given before surgery usually causes this to happen.

2. The medicine which was used to put the patient to sleep will be acting in the patient's body for the next twenty-four (24) hours, so the patient might feel a little sleepy; this feeling will slowly wear off. Because the medicine is still in the patient's system, for the next twenty-four hours the adult patient should not:
   A. drive a car, operate machinery, or power tools,
   B. drink any alcoholic drinks (not even beer), or
   C. make any important decision, such as sign important papers.

3. The patient may have some pain. A prescription for pain may be given by the doctor. This should be taken as directed; and if it does not decrease the pain, contact the patient's doctor. If the doctor does not prescribe anything for pain, the patient may take a non-prescription, non-aspirin pain medication which can be purchased at the drugstore. Please follow the directions on the label.

4. The patient may eat anything, but it is better to start with liquids; such as, water or juice, then soup and crackers, and gradually work up to solid foods. Babies may be fed their milk as soon as they are hungry.

5. The patient is not expected to have any fever; but if the patient does feel warm after today, take his/her temperature. If the temperature is 101 degrees, or higher call the patient's doctor.

6. We strongly suggest that a responsible adult be with the patient for the rest of the day and also during the night for the patient's protection and safety.

7. If any questions arise, call the patient's doctor. If unable to reach the patient's doctor, please feel free to call outpatient surgery. During the day (5 am-5 pm) Monday through Friday, you may call 208-322-7575. At night or on weekends, call the Emergency Department at 208-322-7570.

LBaker, RN	11-26-91		Shelly Hall	11/26/91	
Nurse Signature	Date	Time	Patient Signature	Date	Time

8. The patient has an app0intment with Dr. _____

   Date: _____   Time: _____

9. Call Doctor _____ to make an app0intment.

   Special Instructions: _____ Follow verbal instructions from Dr. Patheal_____

   _____

Nurse Signature	Date	Time	Patient Signature	Date	Time

Outpatient Surgery Discharge Instructions

Idaho Memorial Hospital
876 Memory Ln, Anywhere, ID 83776
(208) 378-5555
OR-2

SURGERY SUPPLY CHARGE CARD

08-26-xx

LABEL	LABEL	LABEL	LABEL
Oximeter			
Dinamap			

Idaho Memorial Hospital
876 Memory Lane, Anywhere, ID 83776
(208) 378-5555

	Maiden Name	Date of Birth	Record Number	Date of Admission	Time of Admission
Patient Name Studabaker, Ezekiel		11/7/xx	420781	09/03/xx	1100
	Social Security Number 515-56-3372	**Gender** M	**Race** C	**Marital Status** M	**Date of Discharge** 09/03/xx	**Time of Discharge** 1600
Patient Address 457 Violet Way Ontario, ID 83798					

Patient Telephone Number 208 355-3565	**Occupation** Retired		**Birthplace** ID	**Religion** Prot	**Length of Stay** 1	**Room Number** IP
Primary Insurer Blue Shield	**Policy and Group Number** 56265302		**Secondary Insurer** NA		**Policy Number** NA	**Group Number** NA
Guarantor Name Same	**Guarantor Relationship** self		**Next of Kin Name** Studabaker, Patrick			**Relationship** son
Guarantor Address 457 Violet Way Ontario, ID 83798	**Guarantor Telephone** 208 355-3565		**Next of Kin Address** 457 Violet Way Ontario, ID 83798			**Telephone** 208 355-3565
Admitting Physician Dr. Tim Tomlinson	**Service Type** OPS		**Admit Type** OPS	**Admitted From** Home	**Address** 457 Violet Way Ontario, ID 83798	**Telephone** 208 355-3565

Attending Physician Dr. Tim Tomlinson	**Attending Physician UPIN** 65524	**Admission Diagnosis** Cancer

Diagnoses and Procedures

Principle Diagnoses			**ICD-9-CM Code**
Bilateral inguinal masses			

Secondary Diagnoses			
Right hydrocele			

Principle Procedure			
Bilateral inguinal hernia and right hydrocelectomy			

Secondary Procedure			

210

Idaho Memorial Hospital
876 Memory Lane, Anywhere, ID 83776
(208) 378-5555

HISTORY AND PHYSICAL

PATIENT: Studabaker, Ezekiel

ROOM#:   106

ADMIT DATE: 09/03/XX

PHYSICIAN: Tim Tomlinson, M.D.

CHIEF COMPLAINT: Bilateral inguinal masses.

HISTORY OF PRESENT ILLNESS: This is a 72-year-old white male who noticed a left inguinal mass about one year ago. It recently has been increasing in size. He noticed a right inguinal mass about six months ago. They are not really painful but they get uncomfortable when he is up and active.

PAST HISTORY:
CURRENT MEDS: Cardura 4 mg, half-tablet once a day. Aspirin 325 mg. once a day.
ALLERGIES: None.
SURGERIES: Hemorrhoidectomy about 25 years ago. Nasal polypectomy. He also had tendon repair of the right middle finger when he tore the tendon and also a cut to, I believe, the index finger, which I believe is still a little bit numb. He has had several skin cancers removed from his face.
MEDICAL ILLNESS: BPH in the past, treated with Cardura for the last several years. No other serious medical problems except possibly a suspected heart attack in about 19XX. He had a problem with ear infections in about 19XX.

SOCIAL HISTORY: Patient is retired. He is married and does not use alcohol or tobacco.

FAMILY HISTORY: Fairly unremarkable. Father died at age of 86 of old age. Mother died at age 42 of pneumonia. A brother died of an accident at the age of 21 and another died at the age of 26 of an unknown cause. One sister died at age of 71 of emphysema, one died of cancer of unknown kind at the age of 81. He has a brother, age 76, who has some arthritis. Sister, age 79, who is in good health.

REVIEW OF SYSTEMS: He wears glasses. He wears a hearing aid on the left side. There is a hole in his right ear drum and has no hearing there. He wears partial dentures. He has had no sense of smell since the nasal polyps were removed in the 60's. He has some occasional shortness of breath when he is real active. He does have nocturia x3 and occasionally difficulty starting his stream. He states these symptoms have improved slightly and have not gotten worse since he started on the Cardura.

PHYSICAL EXAM:
GENERAL: Alert white male in no acute distress.
HEENT: Remarkable for hearing aid in place on the left. Decreased hearing on the right. I cannot see his ear drum real clearly. Several missing teeth. Partial denture in place. Cataract formation on both eyes (the patient is seeing an eye doctor and is planning on having cataract surgery in the near future).
NECK: The trachea is in midline, thyroid is not enlarged. Carotids are equal. No adenopathy noted.

(continued)

CHEST:	Lungs are clear.
HEART:	Regular rate and rhythm.
BREASTS:	No breast enlargement. No lymphadenopathy.
ABDOMEN:	Soft. Bowel sounds are active. There is a reducible left inguinal mass, a smaller reducible right inguinal mass. No other masses or megaly. Bowel sounds are active.
EXTREM:	Full range of motion. All pulses present. Scars on finger of his right hand.
GU:	Normal male. Both testes descended. There is a hydrocele on the right side. This transilluminates and is about 3 cm. in size.
RECTAL:	No masses or tenderness. Prostate is smooth, no particularly enlarged. Stool is guaiac negative.
NEURO:	Grossly normal.
SKIN:	Normal color and turgor.

ADMISSION DIAGNOSIS:

1. Bilateral inguinal hernia.
2. Right hydrocele.

PLAN:

1. Plan to do bilateral inguinal hernia and right hydrocelectomy today as an outpatient. The procedure and risks involved were explained to the patient and he is agreeable to the surgery.

TCT/shc
08/28

TTomlinson, MD

Tim Tomlinson, M.D.

HISTORY AND PHYSICAL

Idaho Memorial Hospital
876 Memory Lane, Anywhere, ID 83776
(208) 378-5555

OPERATIVE REPORT

PATIENT: Studabaker, Ezekiel

ROOM#: 106

ADMIT DATE: 09/03/XX

SURGEON: Jack Ewart, D.O.

PREOPERATIVE DIAGNOSIS: Bilateral inguinal hernia, right hydrocele.
POSTOPERATIVE DIAGNOSIS: Bilateral inguinal hernia, right hydrocele.

PROCEDURE DONE: Bilateral inguinal hernia repair, right hydrocelectomy.

SURGEON: Ewart.
ANESTHESIA: Local plus monitored anesthesia care.
ESTIMATED BLOOD LOSS: 10 cc.
IV FLUIDS: 550 cc lactated Ringer's.

SUMMARY OF THE PROCEDURE: The patient was placed on the operating table in a supine position. The abdomen was prepped with Betadine gel and draped in the usual fashion for bilateral inguinal hernia repair. The right side was done first. Local anesthesia was achieved by means of injection of local anesthetic consisting of one part 1% Xylocaine with epinephrine and one part 0.5% Marcaine with epinephrine. This was injected into the skin, subcutaneous tissue, and fascial planes. A total of 32 cc was used throughout the procedure. The patient also received 112 mg of Ketamine and 500 mg of Diprivan IV during the procedure for sedation as per anesthesia. Once local anesthesia was achieved on the right, a skin incision was made through skin and subcutaneous tissue down to the external oblique. Bleeding was controlled by means of the Bovie. External oblique was divided in the direction of its fibers down to the external ring. The cord was mobilized. Exploration of the cord revealed a small indirect sac. This was dissected free from the cord structures up to the level of the internal ring, suture ligated there and removed. The stump of the hernia sac was allowed to retract as there was no bleeding. Following this the testicle was brought up and the hydrocele was dissected free from its attachments to the testicle with blunt and sharp dissection. No significant bleeding was encountered. The hydrocele was sent to pathology along with the hernia sac. The testicle and epididymis were then replaced back in the scrotum in the anatomic position. A Shouldice type repair was done then using a 0 Prolene suture starting at the level of the symphysis pubis and running up to the level of the internal ring tightening the internal ring. This was used to imbricate the transversalis fascia. It was run back down and tied to itself further imbricating the transversalis fascia. A second 0 Prolene suture was used to imbricate not only the transversalis fascia but also the shelving edge and the internal oblique. It was run up to the level of the internal ring and run back down and tied to itself. A small relaxing incision was made on the anterior rectus fascia. Following this the wound was painted with Betadine solution, hemostasis having been achieved. The ilioinguinal nerve was not clearly identified at any point. The external oblique was approximated with running 3-0 Vicryl suture. Subcutaneous tissue was approximated with interrupted 3-0 Vicryl. Following this a sponge with Betadine solution was placed on top of the wound and attention switched to the left side. After local anesthesia was achieved, a skin incision was made through the skin and subcutaneous tissue down to the external oblique. Bleeding was controlled by means of the Bovie. External oblique was divided in the direction of its fibers down to the external ring. The cord was mobilized. The ilioinguinal nerve was identified and retracted medially. The patient was noted to have some prominence of his femoral artery consistent perhaps with a small femoral artery aneurysm. Inspection of the cord revealed a rather larger thick indirect sac. This was dissected free up to the level of the internal ring and entered. No intra-abdominal contents were noted. This was then twisted and suture ligated at the level of the internal ring and sent to pathology. The stump was allowed to retract after there was no bleeding noted. Following this a Shouldice type repair was done using a 0 Prolene suture starting at the level of the symphysis pubis, anchored there and run up to the level of the internal ring imbricating the transversalis fascia. It was used to tighten the internal ring. It was run back down and tied to itself, further imbricating not only the transversalis fascia but also the

(continued)

shelving edge and the internal oblique. It was run up to the level of the internal ring and run back down and tied to itself. There was no undue tension noted on the repair. Hemostasis having been achieved the wound was painted with Betadine solution. The cord and the ilioinguinal nerve were replaced in the anatomic position. The external oblique was approximated with a running 3-0 Vicryl suture. Subcutaneous tissue was approximated with interrupted 3-0 Vicryl. Following this both skin incisions were approximated with running 3-0 Dexon subcuticular suture. Tega-derm dressings were applied. Sponge count and instrument count were correct. The patient tolerated the procedure well and left the Operating Room in good condition.

TCT/shc
09/03

Jck Ewart, DO

Jack Ewart, D.O.

OPERATIVE REPORT

Idaho Memorial Hospital
876 Memory Lane, Anywhere, ID 83776
(208) 378-5555

TISSUE REPORT

PATIENT: Studabaker, Ezekiel R.

DATE: 09/03/XX

SEX – AGE: M – 72   DOB: 11/07/XX

DOCTOR: Tomlinson, Ewart

ORIGIN: ABDOMEN

TISSUE: Bilateral hernia sac, right hydrocele
                 BPH

HISTORY: Left sac tagged

GROSS: The specimen consists of a 40 × 30 × 15 mm cystic fragment of tissue filled with clear fluid and being multiloculated at one edge. Also received is a 20 × 3 × 2 mm fragment of membranous grey tan tissue as well as a 30 × 12 × 5 mm membranous fragment of grey tan tissue with some attached nodular brown to tan tissue containing suture, the latter fragment inked and representative portions submitted in one block.

MICROSCOPIC: DONE

DIAGNOSIS: SPERMATOCELE, RIGHT
                   HERNIA SACS, INGUINAL, BILATERAL

Chris Shaw, M.D

Chris Shaw, M.D.

CS:shc

CO:9
Code A
9 5 00/1117
CONSTULATION: TM ( )   GE ( )   CO ( )   FF ( )

FILE COPY

Idaho Memorial Hospital
876 Memory Lane, Anywhere, ID 83776
(208) 378-5555

Patient Name	Maiden Name	Date of Birth	Record Number	Date of Admission	Time of Admission
Wilson, Nora	Fields	04/20/xx	564930	03/25/xx	1400
Patient Address	**Social Security Number**	**Gender**	**Marital Status**	**Date of Discharge**	**Time of Discharge**
1052 W. Sapphire Way #456 Kenora, Id	518-42-3265	F	C	M	03/27/xx	1400
Patient Telephone No.	**Occupation**		**Birthplace**	**Religion**	**Length of Stay**	**Room Number**
208-654-4563	retired		ID	Prot	2	
Primary Insurer	**Policy and Group Number**		**Secondary Insurer**		**Policy Number**	**Group Number**
Medicare Non-DRG	51916426 3A		NA		NA	NA
Guarantor Name	**Guarantor Relationship**		**Next of Kin Name**			**Relationship**
Self			Olga Fried			Dtr
Guarantor Address	**Guarantor Telephone**		**Next of Kin Address**			**Telephone**
			6532 Macentire Pl, Kenora, ID 83685			208 855-3245
Admitting Physician	**Service Type**		**Admit Type**	**Admitted From**	**Address**	**Telephone**
Dr. Daniel Lacl	ER		OBS	Home		
Attending Physician	**Attending Physician UPIN**		**Admission Diagnosis**			
Dr. Daniel S. Lacl	59524		Acute bronchitis			

Diagnoses and Procedures ICD-9-CM

Principle Diagnoses Code

Acute bronchitis superimposed on CAD

Secondary Diagnoses

History of intermittent vaginal bleeding and spotting during the past year.

Principle Procedure

Secondary Procedure

Total Charges: $

DISCHARGE SUMMARY

ADMISSION DATE: 3-25-XX

DISCHARGE DATE: 3-27-XX

This 76-year-old patient is in the IMH 3-25 to 3-27. She was admitted because of progressive cough of 2 weeks' duration which had become worse. This morning she had an episode where she became clammy, white, diaphoretic and had possible syncope. This was associated with severe coughing. She's also had severe fatigue. Her usual medications are Zantac, Cardizem and Maxzide. Recently she's had fatigue and insomnia. She has been unable to take adequate fluids the last 24 hours. She has had an intermittent vaginal show for the past year.

Evaluation in the emergency room was done. Chest X-ray showed mild cardiomegaly. No definite pulmonary infiltration was identified. A small irregularity or possible fracture of the external surface of the pacemaker lead was identified. Review of previous films indicates that this has been present for about 3 or 4 years.

The patient was hospitalized. Studies were done. She was placed on Cipro 500 bid. She improved in the respect that she was able to eat, her color improved. She had minimal sputum and felt better. Her low grade fever reduced. IVs were given to rehydrate the patient. Telemetry throughout this period of time showed normal pacemaker function. She had had pacemaker evaluation at her recent hospitalization which was normal. She continued to have a dry cough and a few minimal basilar rales.

LABORATORY STUDIES: Cultures and sensitivity of the sputum were negative. White count 15.7, nucleated neutrophils 96, hematocrit 40. Urinalysis normal.

The patient improved in a limited manner as described above. The cold agglutinin study is pending.

The patient will be discharged on Cipro 0.5 #10 1 bid, continue with her Cardizem 30 mg tid, Zantac prn, 1 of her ferrous sulfate tablets daily. She has been on Maxzide in the past. Her blood pressure has been normal in the hospital and she has not developed edema. We will defer Maxzide at this time.

FINAL DIAGNOSIS:

1. Upper respiratory infection with severe bronchitis.
2. Arteriosclerotic heart disease, pacemaker, atrial fibrillation in the past. No definite evidence of pacemaker malfunction.

PLAN:

1. Will continue medicines above.
2. Will place patient on 24-hour Holter to identify any possible malfunction.

Daniel Lacl
_____
Daniel S. Lacl, M.D.

DSL/shc
3-27/3-28-xx
#1
cc: office

Idaho Memorial Hospital
876 Memory Lane, Anywhere, ID 83776
(208) 378-5555

HISTORY & PHYSICAL

ADMISSION DATE: 3-25-XX

This 76-year-old patient has had progressive intermittent cough for 2 weeks which is gradually becoming worse in spite of home therapy for an upper respiratory infection. She has used anti-inflammatories and cough syrup. This morning this became severe, she became clammy. The daughter states she was pasty and white and severely diaphoretic and a few minutes later she found the patient on the floor and unconscious. She has also had severe fatigue during the past few days.

Her usual medication are Zantac, Cardizem and Maxzide. She has not been taking the Maxzide daily. More recently she has had fatigue and insomnia.

PAST HISTORY: See previous records. These are not available at this time.

The patient states she has taken minimal intake for the past 24 hours. She denies other symptoms.

PHYSICAL EXAMINATION: The patient is a pale, acutely ill adult white female who looks pale, weak and sick.

HEAD & NECK: Normal.
EARS, NOSE & THROAT: Unremarkable.
LUNGS: Clear to P&A. A few rales are heard which are inconstant.
HEART TONES: Normal. Rhythm is regular.
ABDOMEN: Soft without masses. Femoral pulses are normal.
BACK: Normal. Renal percussion tenderness is absent.
EXTREMITIES: Normal. Reflexes are physiologic. Edema is absent.
RECTAL & PELVIC: Were not done.

ADDENDUM: Patient states she has been having intermittent vaginal flowing for the past year.

IMPRESSION:

1. Acute bronchitis superimposed on CAD.
2. History of intermittent vaginal bleeding and spotting during the past year.

PLAN: See orders.

Daniel Lacl
_____
Daniel S. Lacl, M.D.

DSL:shc
3-25/3-26-xx
#2
cc: office

Idaho Memorial Hospital
876 Memory Lane, Anywhere, ID 83776
(208) 378-5555

Nursing Notes

Date: 3-25-XX   Time: 14:00

Time	BP	T	P	R	Nursing Notes:
					Brief History: Today she states she almost "blacked out" several times. About an hour ago she became real disphoretic & pale. C/o some pain upper back. States she has had a dry nonproductive cough for past 2 weeks. Dyspnea Present Meds: Zantac, Cardizem, Maxzide Past Illnesses: Cardiac Allergies: Morphine, Sulfa, PCN, Codeine
200	122/61	97.8	73	20	CXR, CBC
					Sputum- gram stain & culture
					UA
					Blood culture × 3½ hr apart
200					Monitor lead, O2 wl.
230					To Xray, retn @ 240
					UA sent ------ BAllee, LPN
1600					In fair condition for D/C per W/C
					Daniel Lacl —————————— Daniel S. Lacl, M.D

Nursing Notes

Idaho Memorial Hospital
876 Memory Lane, Anywhere, ID 83776
(208) 378-5555

3/25/XX   14:41:49   Dr. Risher and Dr. Narrisog
540660   OPR   208-432-0880 EXT 6423

DOB: 03-42-XX   SEX: F
LAST NAME: Wilson   LOCATION: ER
FIRST NAME: Nora   PHYSICIAN: D. LACL
MED. REC # 8407850   DATE & TIME: 03-25-XX 14:20
AGE: 76

ID: 89662238384	WBC	15.7 H			RBC 4.27
SWALLOW		%	#		HGB 13.8
	NE	96.6 H	15.2	H	HCT 40.5
	LY	2.7 L	0.4	L	MCV 94.8
DATE: 3/25/XX	MO	0.4	0.1		MCH 32.3
TIME: 14:35:57	EO	0.3	0.0		MCHC 34.0
CASS/POS 001703	BA	0.0	0.0		RDW 12.3

Abnormal WBC Pop   PLT 156
Normal RBC Pop   MPV 8.3
Normal PLT Pop

SUSPECT FLAGS:

Imm Grans/Bends
_____WBC_____RBC_____PLT_____

DEFINITE PLAGS:

Leukocytosis
Neutrophilia%
Neutrophilia #
Neutrophilia #
Lymphopenia%
Lymphopenia #

FOR MANUAL

DIFFERENTIAL		RBC MORPHOLOGY	
SEGS	79	NORMAL	
BANDS	16	ROULEAUX	
LYMPHS	1	ANISOCYTOSIS	
MONOS	4	MICROCYTOSIS	
EOS		MACROCYTOSIS	
BASOS		HYPOCHROMA	
METAS		POLYCHROMASIA	
MYELOS		POIXILOCYTOSIS	
ATYP.LYMPH'S		ELLIPTOCYTES	
DOHLE BODIES		DACRYOCYTES	
ABS GRANULO	4.8	CODOCYTES	
ASS. LYMPH	16	ACANTHOCYTES	
DATE DONE	TECH		
3/25/XX	DL		

Idaho Memorial Hospital
876 Memory Ln, Anywhere, ID 83776
(208) 378-5555

EXAM: Chest

HISTORY: Syncopal episode

CHEST:

There is mild cardiomegaly. The patient has a permanent cardiac pacemaker device and I'm suspicious that one of the leads is broken just above the pacemaker as it enters the sheath. Previous film done in February shows the same appearance of the lead. No other change in the pacemaker. The lungs are clear. Hemidiaphragms are normal.

IMPRESSION:

Mild cardiomegaly.? fracture in one of the pacemaker leads.

Brent Buhlard, M.D.
_____
Brent Buhlard, MD
RADIOLOGIST

BBB/shc

Idaho Memorial Hospital
876 Memory Ln, Anywhere, ID 83776
(208) 378-5555

RESPIRATORY CARE OXYGEN RECORD

DIAGNOSIS: ? Bronchitis

DATE/TIME	MODALITY	LPM/FIO$_2$	ON/OFF	RT
3-25 /1800	NO$_2$	2	X / bottle cana	P Spearlock
/ 2300	NO$_2$	2	X/	as
3-26 / 0300	NO$_2$	2	X /	as
/ 0600	NO$_2$	2	X /	as
/ 1100	NO$_2$	2	/ r/h 86	P Spearlock
/ 1500	NO$_2$	2	/X	P Spearlock
/ 1840	NO$_2$	2	/ X	P Spearlock
/ 2300	NO$_2$	2	/ X	as
3-27 / 0300	NO$_2$	2	/ X	as
/ 0600	NO$_2$	2	/ X	as
/ 1100	NN	2	/ X	Jeyn
/ 1500	NN	2	/ X	Jeyn
		Discharged		JJ

NO$_2$ = NASAL OXYGEN
VMO$_2$ = VENTIMASK OXYGEN
MO$_2$ = MASK OXYGEN
TAO$_2$ = TRACH AEROSOL OXYGEN
MHA = MASK HEATED AEROSOL

DIAGNOSTIC IMAGING

Idaho Memorial Hospital
876 Memory Lane, Anywhere, ID 83776
(208) 378-5555

Physician's Orders & Progress Notes

Instructions: Notate progress of case, complications, change in diagnosis, condition on discharge, & instructions to patient.

Date & Time	Orders	X	Date & Time	Progress Notes
3/25	CXR – done in ER Admit Medical 24 hr stay Blood cultures x 3 ½ hour apart, then start Cipro 500 mg Bid. Sputum culture and gram stain T.O Dr D. Lacl *Daniel Lacl* Noted STwitchell, RN			Possible Bronchitis Prog intermittent Cough for 2 wks w/o prog worse. Severe this am, became clammy, pasty white, Diaphoresis, & syncope & on floor. Severe fatigue
3-25-XX 1740	May have diet as tolerated O2 2l NC T.O Dr D. Lacl Noted STwitchell, RN IV 125 ½ NS with 10KCL At 75cc/hr. Old charts please Alternate 1.0 neg hrs from *Daniel Lacl* Noted STwitchell, RN			Cur Rx: Zantac, Cardizem, Maxzide Recently fatigue, insomnia Minimal intake past 24 hours Intermittent Vag show past year *Daniel Lacl*

x = only the prescribed medication may be dispensed.

Physician's Orders   Progress Notes

Idaho Memorial Hospital
876 Memory Lane, Anywhere, ID 83776
(208) 378-5555

Physician's Orders & Progress Notes

Instructions: Notate progress of case, complications, change in diagnosis, condition on discharge, & instructions to patient.

Date & Time	Orders	X	Date & Time	Progress Notes
3/25/xx	Nora to be on Tele to check pacemaker PO order Dr. D Lacl BMuir, LPN 2115 Noted STwitchell, RN -------- Daniel Lacl			
3-26-XX	Bedside humidifier Up fam. Cardizem 30 tid -------- Daniel Lacl Noted G Lambert, LPN 1020		3-26	Dry cough continues Lungs clear Ate a little breakfast. On telemetry re pacemaker ➢ To check for a break in connectivity of pacer pain lead extended cover. Review of prior films—this has been present 3-4 yrs. -------- Daniel Lacl To okay ed FE & Maxzide at present -------- Daniel Lacl

x = only the prescribed medication may be dispensed.

Physician's Orders   Progress Notes

Idaho Memorial Hospital
876 Memory Lane, Anywhere, ID 83776
(208) 378-5555

Physician's Orders & Progress Notes

Instructions: Notate progress of case, complications, change in diagnosis, condition on discharge, & instructions to patient.

Date & Time	Orders	X	Date & Time	Progress Notes
3/27/xx	Cold agglute please Repeat to Mcall office DC IV Faxed repeats of sputum C&S for Dr LSC office ---------- *Daniel Lacl* Release ---------- *Daniel Lacl* *Noted G Lambert, LPN 1000*		3-27	Cough continues, dry. Stronger, eating A few fair brush rales. ---------- *Daniel Lacl* C&S neg thus far Sp culture uncertain thus far. ---------- *Daniel Lacl*

x = only the prescribed medication may be dispensed.

Physician's Orders   Progress Notes

PROBLEM NURSING DIAGNOSIS / EXPECTED OUTCOME		INTERVENTION
SAFETY CHECK: (CALL LIGHT ACCESSIBLE, BED RAILS UP, ETC) checked q1hr HYGIENE: HS cares DIET: SAT		ACTIVITY INTAKE OUTPUT
ALTERATION IN RESP FUNCTION: ASSESSMENT NURSING CARE	SPONTANEOUS VENTILATION PERFORMS NECESS SELF-CARE ROUTINES RESP RATE WNL FOR PT RESP REGULAR/UNLABORED CHEST CLEAR PER AUSCULTATION	BREATH SOUNDS RESP PATTERN/EFFORT/RATE S/S HYPOXIA ADEQUACY OF FLUID BALANCE TDB Q4H WHILE AWAKE & PRN CHARAC/FREQ/EFFECTIVENESS OF COUGH SECRETIONS FOR CHARACTER/ VOLUME
PATIENT SAFETY DEFICITS	WILL REMAIN FREE OF FALLS REMAIN ORIENTED X 3 CALL/REQUEST ASSISTANCE PRN	ASSESS RISK FALLS/INJURY INSTRUCT RE: SAFETY PROTOCOLS EVALUATE ONGOING SAFETY STATUS REORIENT X 3 FALLS PREVENTION PROGRAM SIDERAILS UP PHONE IN REACH BED IN LOW POSITION
KNOWLEDGE DEFICIT: UNIT/ HOSPITAL ORIENTATION	pt/so understand hosp/rout/regim	EXPLAIN VISITING POLICIES TO PT/SO REVIEW NURSING/MEDICAL ROUTINES EXPLAIN PURPOSE/FUNC OF EQUIPMENT REVIEW NURSE CALL SYSTEM IDENTIFY KEY PERSONNEL FOR HELP ORIENT TO UNIT/HOSP FACILITIES PROVIDE PRINTED INFO TO PT/SO
TIME: 1615 T: 99.5 P: 68 R: 20 BP: 96/68		

NURSING CARE PLAN / FLOW (1)

Idaho Memorial Hospital
876 Memory Lane, Anywhere, ID 83776
(208) 378-5555

Nursing Notes

Date: 03/25

Time	BP	T	P	R	
1630					76 y.o. female admitted via wc from ER. States has had weakness, been real Tired & had dry non prod. Cough x2 weeks. States weaker today and "passed out" at home this morning. Was weak, shaky, pale & "clammy" before and after Blacking out. States has been under stress because husband ill & child with cancer. Pt resting quietly – alert & oriented. Very pale with skin warm & dry Denies any chest pain or tightness. States "raspy" feeling in midchest when coughs. Has dry non prod cough. ---------- STwitchell, RN
2200					IV started (L) arm with 20 gauge needle D51/2 NS with 10KCL @ 75cc/h ----------RBendenhall, Rn

Nursing Notes

PROBLEM NURSING DIAGNOSIS / EXPECTED OUTCOME	INTERVENTION
SAFETY CHECK: (CALL LIGHT ACCESSIBLE, BED RAILS UP, ETC) top rails up	3-11 SA^^, checked Q1h ~ RB 3-11 SH, assist PRN ~ RB ACTIVITY: BRP w/ assist
HYGIENE: SH	INTAKE:
DIET: Reg -8 -75% 12-50% 3-11Reg-Din 60%	OUTPUT:

ALTERATION IN RESP FUNCTION: ASSESSMENT NURSING CARE	SPONTANEOUS VENTILATION	BREATH SOUNDS RESP PATTERN/EFFORT/RATE S/S HYPOXIA
	PERFORMS NECESS SELF-CARE ROUTINES RESP RATE WNL FOR PT RESP REGULAR/UNLABORED CHEST CLEAR PER AUSCULTATION	ADEQUACY OF FLUID BALANCE TDB Q4H WHILE AWAKE & PRN SECRETIONS FOR CHARACTER/VOLUME

PATIENT SAFETY DEFICITS	WILL REMAIN FREE OF FALLS REMAIN ORIENTED X 3 CALL/REQUEST ASSISTANCE PRN	ASSESS RISK FALLS/INJURY INSTRUCT RE: SAFETY PROTOCOLS EVALUATE ONGOING SAFETY STATUS REORIENT X 3 FALLS PREVENTION PROGRAM SIDERAILS UP PHONE IN REACH BED IN LOW POSITION

K –Hamilton, RN

TIME:	8	16
T:	96	98.2
P:	80	68
R:	16	16
BP:	100/60	110/70

NURSING CARE PLAN / FLOW (1)

DATE: 3/27/XX MEDICAL DIAGNOSIS_____

PROBLEM NURSING DIAGNOSIS / EXPECTED OUTCOME		INTERVENTION
SAFETY CHECK: (CALL LIGHT ACCESSIBLE, BED RAILS UP, ETC) low rails up		
		ACTIVITY: up ad lib
HYGIENE: S		INTAKE:
DIET: Reg		OUTPUT:
KNOWLEDGE DEFICIT SELF CARE/ DISCHARGE REGIMEN 45	DEMONS ABILITY SAFELY PERFORM ADL'S DEMONS ABILITY SAFELY TAKE MEDS PT/SO IDENT S/S REQUIRING MED CARE CAUSE/SELF-HELP TECH: RELIEF-PREVENT	ASSESS POTENT SAFETY DEFICITS INSTRCT RE: SAFTY HAZRD IN HOME TEACH /REV S/S REQUIR F/U CARE NOTIFY MD OF PTENTIAL SAFTY DEF PULMONARY SELF-CARE ROUTINES S/S INFECTION MEDICATION REGIMEN: ACTIVITY REGIMEN: FLUID/DIET REGIMEN: SELF-CARE TECH
ALTERATION IN RESP FUNCTION: ASSESSMENT NURSING CARE 1	SPONTANEOUS VENTILATION PERFORMS NECESS SELF-CARE ROUTINES RESP RATE WNL FOR PT RESP REGULAR/UNLABORED CHEST CLEAR PER AUSCULTATION	BREATH SOUNDS RESP PATTERN/EFFORT/RATE S/S HYPOXIA ADEQUACY OF FLUID BALANCE TDB Q4H WHILE AWAKE & PRN CHAR/FREQ/EFFECTIVENESS OF COUGH
PATIENT SAFETY DEFICITS 9	WILL REMAIN FREE OF FALLS REMAIN ORIENTED X 3 CALL/REQUEST ASSISTANCE PRN	ASSESS RISK FALLS/INJURY INSTRUCT RE: SAFETY PROTOCOLS EVALUATE ONGOING SAFETY STATUS REORIENT X 3 FALLS PREVENTION PROGRAM SIDERAILS UP PHONE IN REACH BED IN LOW POSITION

K –Hamilton, RN

TIME: 8
T: 98
P: 80
R: 20
BP: 100/70

NURSING CARE PLAN / FLOW (1)

Idaho Memorial Hospital
876 Memory Lane, Anywhere, ID 83776
(208) 378-5555

Nursing Notes

Date: 03/27/XX

Time	BP	T	P	R	
1400					Discharge instructions given, she stated she would follow them. To auto per Amb w/son, by nurse. -------------M Marin, LPN
1100					Instructed to call Dr D Lacl office daily to report progress. Verbalizes understanding of instructions -------------B Surroul, LPN

Idaho Memorial Hospital
876 Memory Lane, Anywhere, ID 83776
(208) 378-5555

Discharge Instructions

DIET: _____ Regular _____

_____

_____

ACTIVITY: _____ as tolerated _____

_____

_____

MEDICATIONS: _____

Rocephin 30   3× a day.

Cifras 0.5   one 2× a day.

Tristan if needed

lone iron daily

_____

_____

SPECIAL INSTRUCTIONS: _____ To office for Holter. _____

_____

_____

_____

FOLLOW UP APPOINTMENT: _____

_____

_____

I have read and understand the above instructions. I also understand that if any problem arises I should contact my physician.

_____*Nora Wilson*_____

SIGNATURE OF PATIENT OR RESPONSIBLE PARTY

COMMENT: (Regarding patient's ability to verbalize or demonstrate his/her understanding of instructions) <u>able to understand her instructions and verbalize them</u>

_____*SBall*_____

SIGNATURE OF PHYSICIAN OR NURSE

DATE: _____ 3/27/XX _____

Nursing Notes

Idaho Memorial Hospital
876 Memory Lane, Anywhere, ID 83776
(208) 378-5555

Patient Name	Maiden Name	Date of Birth	Record Number	Date of Admission	Time of Admission
Young, Paul		06/26/xx	837155	03/25/xx	0830

Social Security Number	Gender	Race	Marital Status	Date of Discharge	Time of Discharge
587-36-4569	M	C	W	04/01/XX	1600

Patient Address	Birthplace	Religion	Length of Stay	Room Number
647 Orchard Way Commerce, ID 86587	ID	Prot	8	314

Patient Telephone Number	Occupation	Secondary Insurer	Policy Number	Group Number
208 569-1236	retired	NA	NA	NA

Primary Insurer	Policy and Group Number
Medicare	56243302A

Guarantor Name	Guarantor Relationship	Next of Kin Name	Relationship
Young, Jason	son	Young, Jason	Son

Guarantor Address	Guarantor Telephone	Next of Kin Address	Telephone
647 Orchard Way Commerce, ID 86587	208 569-1236	647 Orchard Way Commerce, ID 86587	208 569-1236

Admitting Physician	Service Type	Admit Type	Admitted From	Address	Telephone
Dr. Nancy Squires	OPS	IP	Home	647 Orchard Way Commerce, ID 86587	208 569-1236

Attending Physician	Attending Physician UPIN	Admission Diagnosis
Dr. Patrick Manwise	83604	Cervical thoracic spine fractures

Diagnoses and Procedures

	ICD-9-CM Code
Principle Diagnoses	
Multiple laminar fractures posterior spine	
Secondary Diagnoses	
Fracture posterior spinous process C7, T1, T2, and T3.	
Principle Procedure	
local in situ fusion C7-T1, T1-T2, T2-T3, T3-T4, T4-T5 (6 levels).	
Secondary Procedure	
Harvesting of left iliac posterior autologous bone graft for fusion	

Total Charges:	$12499.

Idaho Memorial Hospital
876 Memory Ln, Anywhere, ID 83776
(208) 378-5555

Hospital #789456

DISCHARGE/TRANSFER SUMMARY:

DATE OF TRANSFER/ADMISSION ORTHOPEDIC SERVICES: 3/25/XX
DATE OF DISCHARGE/TRANSFER REHAB SERVICES: 4/1/XX

DIAGNOSIS:

1. Multiple laminar fractures posterior spine.
2. Fracture posterior spinous process C7, T1, T2, and T3.
3. Jump locked impacted facet T2-T3 left.
4. Fractured facet T3-T4 bilateral.
5. Fracture posterior lamina C7, T1, T2, and T3 on right side only.
6. Neurologically intact individual.
7. Multiple rib fractures secondary to crush syndrome.
8. Mild exogenous obesity.

OPERATIONS & DIAGNOSTIC PROCEDURES PERFORMED:

1. Exploration of cervical thoracic spinal fractures as noted above with anticipation of internal fixation with rods & sublaminar wire fixation which was aborted and local in situ fusion C7-T1, T1-T2, T2-T3, T3-T4, T4-T5 (6 levels).
2. Harvesting of left iliac posterior autologous bone graft for fusion.

OPERATOR: Dr. Manwise, Dr. Deery
CONSULTANTS: None.

LABORATORY DATA:
SMAC 22 3/29/XX, glucose 94, BUN 11, slight elevation of alk phos 180, all other parameters normal. Electrolytes 138, sodium and potassium 3.7. Electrolytes remained normal throughout postoperative hospitalization. On 3/26/XX, glucose 161 with IV in place. BUN 17, slight elevation alk phos at 236, sodium 134. Postoperative hematocrit stabilized in the mid low 30 to upper 20 area and on 3/26/XX, hematocrit 29, hemoglobin 9.9.

Baseline room air arterial blood gas pH 7.44, PCO_2 36, PO_2 131, O_2 saturation 95.

The patient was prophylactically anticoagulated and on 4/1/XX had a protime of 17.5. The patient was given 2 units of homologous blood transfusion postoperatively for a crit that was documented down to 25 on 3/27/XX, with a WBC of 10,300.

A single x-ray was obtained with hospitalization 3/25/XX, lateral review localizing the posterior spinous processes for appropriate operative approach.

HOSPITAL COURSE:

60-year-old male who was thrown from car the first week of March. Initially seen in Twin Falls, Cassia County. Transferred to XXXX rehabilitation unit under the care of Dr. Bekolmann and Dr. Warano. Dr. Bacon was asked to see the patient in consultation along with Dr. Manwise who felt that the patient sustained a relatively unstable fracture subluxation of thoracic spine with a 50% compression fracture T4 by X-ray in addition to 50% anterior subluxation T3 on T4 by outside films. Preoperative CT scans were reperformed and compared to those obtained in Twin Falls. Fractures were not fully visualized on either of the two CT scans and we were quite frankly surprised to see the multiple fractures at the time of the exploration of the thoracic spine at the time of surgery. The multiple fractures and laminar instabilities made intervention with internal fixation virtually impossible with stabilization of the spine with sublaminar technique or hook technique we would have had to hooked into C6 with either sublaminar wire or Harrington hook and we did not feel comfortable doing so. Therefore, we felt that an onlay spinal fusion and the treatment of an external orthosis was best indicated based upon the multiple fractures and fractures of the posterior spinous processes and

(continued)

laminar fractures, facet fractures. The patient did exhibit a fracture impaction subluxation of a T2-T3 facet not appreciated on preoperative CAT scans x2 and because of this instability we considered taking down the facet and relocating this impacted jump locked facet without fracture but we did not feel comfortable doing so because the patient was neurologically intact and we essentially fused it in situ. The patient's postoperative course was unremarkable. Morkylo brace shop was employed to manufacture a body shell with SOMI neck extension. The patient was progressively mobilized to a point of comfort and independence and will be transferred back to the rehab unit for progressive rehabilitation and for home disposition and for further anticoagulation by the rehabilitation specialist on 4/1/XX.

His orthopedic care was stable and he did quite fine with surgery.

DISABILITY: Estimated 1 year 3/25/XX through 3/25/XX

I will see him back in the office in approximately a month for reassessment. Sutures will be removed on the Rehabilitation Unit in the back and the hip area prior to his discharge.

Prior to his transfer back to the rehabilitation unit he was started on prophylactic anticoagulation. He was initially treated with minidose Heparin, TED stockings, pneumatic boots, and aspirin containing compounds. These were essentially discontinued when prothrombin times were adequate and transfer prothrombin time on 4/1/XX, 17.1 seconds after initial loading doses of Coumadin.

RESULT OF TREATMENT: Improved.
COMPLICATIONS: None.

Patrick Manwise
_____
Patrick B. Manwise, M.D.

PBM: shc
4/2-3/XX
#1
CC: Office
     Dr. Deery
     Dr. Bekolmann
     Dr. Warano

Idaho Memorial Hospital
876 Memory Ln, Anywhere, ID 83776
(208) 378-5555

Hospital #789456

CONSULTATION REPORT

DATE: 3-25-xx

PRESENT ILLNESS: This is a 60-year-old male who apparently was involved in a single car rollover accident sustaining what appears to be a complicated fracture involving compression fracture of T2 and T3 by recent x-rays.

In addition he appears to have jump locked impacted facets at T2-T3. He neurologically is intact. I was asked by Dr. Rowona to see him in medical consultation, that consultation should be reviewed.

We feel that his lower cervical spine and upper thoracic spine has a significant potential of instability and fell that he is best served at this time with a thoracolumbar orthosis and cervical extension. In addition, I would recommend instrumentation or at least spine fusion of his affected areas to minimize further difficulty or neurologic deficit.

The patient is a laborer, but is reasonably cognizant.

The patient is otherwise in reasonably good health, does smoke 1-1/2 pack a day.

He denies any allergies, denies any significant prior injuries as well.

Because of his potential instability, I do recommend strongly that fusion be proceeded with and I have asked Dr. Deery to see him in medical evaluation as well for his neurologic assessment. I can demonstrate no evidence of any neurologic damage or deficit.

By preoperative x-rays it appears that he has a fracture subluxation T3- T4 with 80% compression fracture of T4 with retropulsion of vertebral fragments into the spinal canal by tomogram.

In addition it would appear that he has fractured the left pedicle of T3 and fractured the right lamina of T3 indicating a significant probability of instability.

IMPRESSION:
1. Cervical thoracic spine fractures indicated above with potential potentially unstable T3-T4 with 80% subluxation T3 on T4 without significant neurologic compromise or obvious neurologic deficit.

DISPOSITION: I have discussed with the patient in detail the options and care. I would strongly recommend that this be fused and stabilized. If we can wire the vertebral bodies together, even place Harrington fixation rods, this should be done.

If nothing else, then an external orthosis utilizing a cervical thoracic orthosis should be considered for stabilization. I believe the patient understands the potential instability of his fracture and because of his livelihood as a laborer, he wishes to proceed with operative intervention and stabilization and consents to utilization of an external orthosis for six months or so postoperatively. I have been very blunt, frank and straightforward with the patient indicating to him the options and alternative methods of care and I do believe that he wishes to proceed with operative intervention on an elective basis.

I will ask if Dr. Deery will assist in surgery and neurologic assessment as well.

The patient consents to this as well.

Patrick Manwise
_____
Patrick B. Manwise, M.D.

PBM/shc
8-4/8-6-xx
PM805I
CC: Office

Idaho Memorial Hospital
876 Memory Ln, Anywhere, ID 83776
(208) 378-5555

Hospital #789456

OPERATIVE NOTE

DATE OF PROCEDURE: 3-25-xx

PREOPERATIVE DIAGNOSIS:
1. Fracture subluxation T3-T4 with 80% compression fracture of T4 with some retropulsion of vertebral elements into spinal canal.
2. Fracture of left pedicle T3 left, fracture right lamina T3.

POSTOPERATIVE DIAGNOSIS:
1. Considerably different from the above with fractures of posterior spinous processes of C7, T1, T2 and T3 with associated laminar fractures C7, T1, T2, T3.
2. Fracture of T3 facet, left.
3. Fracture subluxation with what appears to be impacted jumplocked facet T2-T3 left without gross instability.
4. Fracture of T2 facet, right.

OPERATIONS & DIAGNOSTIC PROCEDURES PERFORMED:
1. Exploration of spinal fracture thoracic spine with fusion C7-T1, T1-T2, T2-T3, T3-T4, T4-T5 levels with only posterolateral spine fusion.
2. Harvesting of left iliac pelvic crest donor bone graft.

(See below for details and explanation why instrumentation could not be utilized.)

OPERATORS:	Drs. Manwise/Deery
ANESTHESIA:	General by endotracheal intubation.
ANESTHESIOLOGIST:	Dr. Fox
ANESTHETIST:	Gufate

INDICATIONS: 60-year-old male who was riding as a passenger in a Subaru in which the driver lost control, the car went off the road and the car flipped and the patient apparently was thrown from the car sustaining multiple bilateral hemi-thorax rib fractures in addition to the spinal fractures as noted.

He was initially hospitalized at Cassia Hospital in Twin Falls, was stabilized and found to have spinal fractures but apparently they were judged to be stable at that place. He was placed in a body brace with a SOMI chin support.

He was mobilized and sent to the Rehabilitation Unit recently for attempted rehabilitation because he found it increasingly difficult to mobilize secondary to his rib and thoracic spine fractures. Because of the concern of potential instability of the thoracic spine, Dr. Bacon was asked to see him in consultation. He recognized the significant potential of instability and I was asked to see the patient on 3-19-xx. My consultation notes should be reviewed.

It appeared that he had, by outside films, a 50% subluxation T3 on T4 with an 80% compression fracture of T4 with a fracture of the left pedicle T3 and a fracture of the right lamina T3.

These appeared to be isolated injuries as best as I could tell to the spine itself. He is brought into surgery for attempted either sub-laminar wiring and rodding and/or Harrington rodding of the thoracic spine for stabilization and rapid mobilization in addition to fusion.

However, when we entered the spine for exploration, the below findings were noted.

Preoperatively the patient was understanding of the risks, complications, technical limitations, the alternative methods of care and the reasons for consideration of stabilization of his spine. We do feel that the spine is potentially significantly unstable and patient really does merit exploration and attempted stabilization to prevent paraplegia. I believe he was understanding of this preoperatively and consented to surgery.

FINDINGS: With exploration of the thoracic spine fracture, very unusual findings were appreciated which essentially prevented the insertion of Harrington rods or sub-laminar wires for Luque type rods. When we explored the spine fracture, we found that the posterior spinous processes from C7, T1, T2, and T3 were all fractured and grossly unstable. In addition, laminar fractures extended down into the base of the transverse processes at all of these levels bilaterally with extension of the laminar fracture into the mid portion of the body of the lamina at C7, T1, T2 and T3 making sub-laminar wiring or even hook fixation virtually impossible. If stabilization were required, we would have had to have hooked under or wired beneath C6 and we did not feel comfortable doing so.

I could not identify any frank subluxation of the spine although there was an impacted jumplocked facet which was not identified on the preoperative CT scans x2 at the T2-T3 level on the left.

This did not appear to be a fracture of the facet but rather simply an impacted jumplocked facet.

Because the patient was neurologically negative and because no significant instability could be appreciated by this by simply pulling on the fracture, we fused this in situ.

We did not feel that significant spinal stability could be achieved by the internal fixation devices as between the spinous processes and the laminar fractures, extensive fusions would have been necessary up into the lower mid cervical spine and to the upper mid thoracic spine. We did not feel comfortable putting internal fixation hardware at these levels, so therefore the spine was fused in situ and we'll go with external fixation immobilization to prevent further spinal instability.

PROCEDURE: Supine position, endotracheal intubation, Foley catheter, pneumatic boots. Very carefully turned to a prone position face down with 3-point tong head supports, Hibbs back frame, pneumatic boots, prophylactic antibiotics 1 gram Ancef and 500 mg Vancomycin.

The neck and back were prepared routinely with shaving and prepping for approximately 25 minutes as the patient could not receive preoperative preparation for the skin on the ward.

Dr. Deery approached the back and exposed the spine while Dr. Manwise obtained the bone graft. Dr. Deery's notes should be reviewed for details.

A curvilinear incision was made about the left iliac crest area going through approximately 3-4 inches of fat and adipose tissue down to the hip area. Bone graft was obtained. The bone was moderately osteoporotic secondary to age and recumbency for 3 weeks.

Cortical cancellous strips were obtained in routine fashion with single thickness graft available. The wounds were irrigated thoroughly, bone wax applied to the raw bleeding cancellous surfaces after adequate bone graft was obtained and a large piece of dry Gelfoam placed in the donor site area.

This was copiously irrigated throughout the procedure with Ancef and saline solution. Two deep Hemovac drains placed in the left iliac wound. The fascia approximated with #1 absorbable interrupted Vicryl, subcutaneous tissues in multiple layers with 2-0 interrupted Vicryl and the skin with stainless steel skin staples.

Attention was then diverted from the hip wound to the neck area where Dr. Manwise and Dr. Deery approached the upper thoracic and low cervical spine and evaluated the spine for internal fixation.

Our preoperative anticipation and assessment had been to fuse from T1 to T5 or 6 utilizing sub-laminar wires and/or Harrington rods and hooks. However, with evaluation of the spine it became apparent that there was no stable element any lower than C6 to which we could utilize sub-laminar wiring or hook fixation. We could not even wire the posterior spinous processes together as they had all been fractured from C7 to T3.

This was an unexpected finding as it had not been evident on our preoperative X-rays or CT scans taken x 2.

We did note the jumplocked facet without fracture at T2-T3 on the left. We evaluated this for possible takedown but because the patient was neurologically intact and dealing with the thoracic spinal canal, I felt that fusion was best indicated in situ because internal fixation could not be obtained if we removed the inferior facet at T3 to reduce the fracture subluxation impaction. Therefore, the spine was cleansed of its posterior fascial attachments. A Cibatome drill was utilized to drill cooling all points with copious irrigation decorticating the posterior elements and an onlay posterior bone graft was performed from C7 to T5 over a 6-level segment.

(continued)

Bone was tamped securely into position. Two deep Hemovac drains inserted in the subfascial plane. The back fascia approximated with #1 interrupted absorbable Vicryl with the drains free. Subcutaneous tissue was approximated with 2-0 absorbable Vicryl and the skin with stainless steel skin staples. Sterile clear plastic Op-Site dressing was applied to the skin and hip areas. Thoracic brace orthotic with a SOMI attachment was reapplied.

The patient was awakened, extubated, and returned to ICU in stable condition with noted complication.

SPONGE, NEEDLE, INSTRUMENT & PADDY COUNT: Correct at termination of procedure.

OPERATIVE TIME: Slightly less than 3 hours.

COMPLICATIONS: None noted.

BLOOD LOSS: Estimated less than 500 cc's between the hip and back areas. No blood replacement was administered. No Solcotrans postoperative auto transfusion was utilized.

With awakening in the recovery area, the patient moved his toes up and down to command without obvious neurologic deficit as the patient had been apparently neurologically intact preoperatively.

Patrick Manwise
_____
Patrick B. Manwise, M.D.

PBM: mb
3-26/3-27-XX
#4
CC: office
     Dr. P. Deery
     Dr. M. Warano
     Dr. G. Bacon
     Dr. J. Kobelmann

Idaho Memorial Hospital
876 Memory Ln, Anywhere, ID 83776
(208) 378-5555

Hospital #789456

CONSENT TO ANESTHESIA

The nature and purpose of anesthesia, possible alternate methods, the risks involved and the possibility of complications have been explained to me. I am aware that the practice of medicine is not an exact science and acknowledge that no guarantee or assurance has been made as to the results that may be obtained.

I understand that all anesthetics involve risk of complications, serious injury to any body part or function, or rarely death from both known and unknown causes. I understand the possibility of damage to my teeth, mouth and voice box during an anesthetic. Nerve damage is possible during general or regional anesthesia.

When you have had anything to eat or drink recently, as with emergency surgery, there is an increased risk of lung complications.

Anesthesia services are directed by an Anesthesiologist. Anesthesia care is provided by Anesthesiologists and Certified Registered Nurse Anesthetists who are approved by the Medical Staff. I consent to the administration of anesthesia and to the use of such anesthetics as may be deemed advisable.

Consent form given to patient to read on   _03/24/xx_   , _8:30 p.m._
                                                            Date   time

Signature of nurse: _Mary Leach, RN_

I have read the above consent.	I read consent to patient because:
X _PAUL YOUNG_	_His glasses are not here_
Signature of patient	reason
Mason Moore	_Mary Leach RN_
witness to signature	signature of reader relationship
_3-24-xx_ _8:30 pm_	_3/24/xx_ _8:35 pm_
date time	date time

If the patient is unable to consent, or is a minor, please complete the following:

Patient (is a minor ___ years of age) is unable to consent because

Consent is made on behalf of the patient by the undersigned relative or legal representative.

I have read the above consent.

_____   _____a.m./p.m._

signature of closest relative or legal guardian   date   time

Idaho Memorial Hospital
876 Memory Ln, Anywhere, ID 83776
(208) 378-5555

CONSENT TO OPERATION

PATIENT: ___Paul Young_____   _____ Age: ___60 yrs_____

Date: ___3/24/xx_____ Time: 1100 _____ Place: Idaho Memorial Hospital

1. I hereby authorize Dr. Manwise_____ and whomever he may designate as his/her assistants, to perform upon ___myself____. The following operations: __ORIF Thoracic spine fx & fusions same___ and in any unforeseen conditions arises in the course of the operation, calling in his judgement for procedures in addition to, or different from, those now contemplated, I further request and authorize him to do whatever he deems advisable.

2. The nature and purpose of the operation, possible alternative methods of treatment, the risks involved, and the possibility of complications have been explained to me. I acknowledge that no guarantee or assurance has been made t the results that may be obtained.

3. I consent to the administration of anesthesia, and to the use of such anesthetics as the attending physician, anesthesiologist, and the hospital staff may deem advisable. I understand that all anesthetics involve risks or complications, serious injury, or rarely, death from both known and unknown causes, and that no guarantees have been made as to the results of the anesthetic.

4. I consent to the disposal, by authorities of Idaho Memorial Hospital, of any tissues or parts which may have been removed.

5. For the purpose of advancing medical and nursing education, I consent to the admittance of the personnel to the operating room.

I CERTIFY THAT I HAVE READ AND FULLY UNDERSTAND THE ABOVE CONSENT TO OPERATION, THAT THE EXPLANATIONS THEREIN REFERRED TO WERE MADE AND THAT ALL BLANKS FOR COMLETION WERE FILLED IN AND INAPPLICABLE PARAGRAPHS, IF ANY, WERE STRICKEN BEFORE I SIGNED.

_____PAUL YOUNG_____
SIGNATURE OF PATIENT

_____
SIGNATURE OF PATIENT'S HUSBAND OR WIFE

When patient is a minor or incompetent to give consent:

_____
SIGNATURE OF PERSON AUTHORIZED TO CONSENT TO PATIENT

_____
RELATIONSHIP TO PATIENT

_____kay Johansen, RN_____
WITNESS

Anesthesia Record

Surgeon Manwise/Deery	Operation T1-T12 ORIF w/fusion	Date 3/25xx	BP 118/78 120/70 Pulse 50 56
Prior Anesthesia 13 maxillary teeth extracted	Family Anes. Hx. Neg	Teeth up-good Lower-front loose	Weight 240# 5-11

Allergies NONE	ETOH: Beer Cig. 2PPD Hepatitis Neg	Transfusions Neg	Laboratory

Medications Neg — Tx x 4 — High GKPO4

Phys Exam Fx Maxilla R, Fx R Clavicle, T3-4 Fx unstable A2 no paralyzation, R AC dislocation, R Rib Fx — EKG ? inf S waves — GRIP

Anes Risk 2 SAB (General) — Other risk explained to patient — some recall — (NPO) — Hct 42.6

RA 7.4/33/62/24/1.9/89

Premedication	Effect X RM Drake, MD	3/25/xx
Neg	Anesthesiologist	Date

Pulse Ox															IV Started	
O2 Sat %	89	92	97	97	99	100	99	99	99	99	98	97	95	97	SAB Lot #	Exp:
ET CO2 mmHg		37	34	36	34	33	34	34	33	33	32	31	30	30	MAC O2	Nasal Mask INS
Temp. C			35^8	35^7	35^4	35^1	35^0	35^1	34^9	34^4	35^0	34^9			OPA NPA	
EKG Lead			NSR	NSR	NSR	NSR	NSR	NSR	NSR	NSR	NSR	NSR	NSR	NSR	Miller	MAC Stylet LTA
O2 Analyzer %			54	50	50	50	50	50	50	84	86	89	89	91	ET Depth 22 cm	Secured IOR Cuff
Position	→	→	→	→	→	→	→	→	→	→	→	→	→	→	C Pressure	Pre-O2 same
TIDAL Vol: cc				860	850	900	950	100	980	950	970	970	920	920		
Rate/min				7	7	6	6	6	5	5	5	5	5	5	To OR #2	
P.I.P. cm/H2O				30	38	38	38	38	40	40	40	39	39	39	Monitors on	
TIME:	130	145	.2.	215	230	245	.3.	315	330	345	.4.	415	430	445	Line Started	

Precordial
Esophageal
SCCA
J.R.
Bain
Eyes
Lube L R
Tape L R
PNS
Arms Padded
L R
Anesthesia Machine # 6

160/160 15/175
EBL 150 – 300

VVVVVVLL
LL
L LL
LL LL
L LL
LL LL
LL LL LL
LL LL LL

1U Autologous blood withdrawn
Moves Legs

Remarks:
1 – Induction & intubation w/o difficulty
2 – Head Positioned
    prone on white frame
3 – Relief w Rodriguiz, CRNA
BG^1 pH 7.44, PCO$_2$ 36, PO$_2$ 131,
HCO$_3$ 25 TOTCO$_2$ 26, B.E. 0.9,
O$_2$ Sats 95, Hbg 12.5
4 –Dr Deery relieving
see pg 2

Remark No:		1	2		3	1	BG^1					4		
O2 L/M		6	6	1	1	1	1	1	1	2	2	2	2	2	2
N2O L/M			1	1	1	1	1	1	1	x	x	x	x	x	x
Foranel			.4	.4	1	1	1	1.5	0.6	0.5	1.2	1.2	1.0	1.5	0.5
Halothane															
Ethrane															
Pentothal				300											
Fentanyl		2.1	1.1				2			1	1		1	2	
Meterlan				2			1gm Ancef								
Anectine				140			1500 Vancomycin								
Tracrium					25										

Post OP Remarks		800 cc
		E.B.I.
	1U removed and	LR4700
RM Drake, MD 3.25.xx	replaced	Total Fluids:
Anesthesiologist Signature Date/Time	RM Drake, MD C. Rodriguez 3/25/xx	
	Anesthesiologist/CRNA Date	

Anesthesia Record

Idaho Memorial Hospital

© 2011 Pearson Education, Inc.

APPENDIX 241

Anesthesia Record

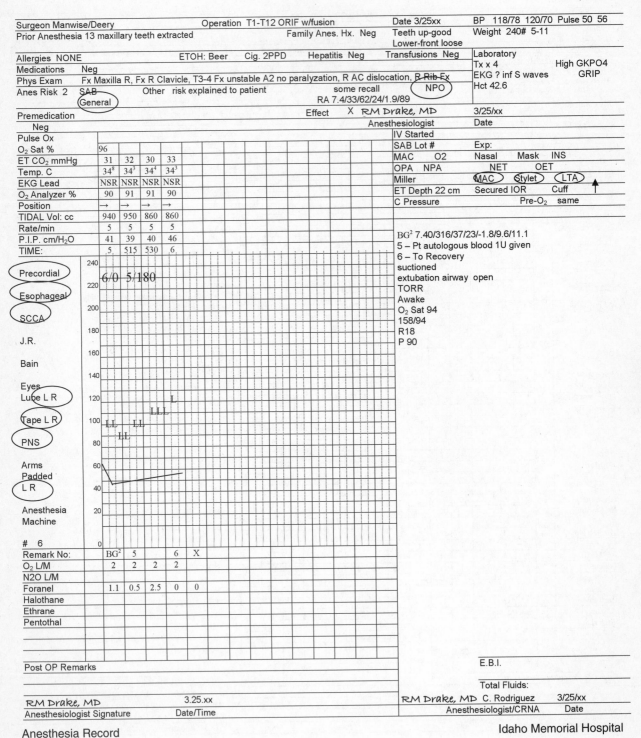

Idaho Memorial
Hospital

Surgeon Manwise/Deery	Operation T1-T12 ORIF w/fusion	Date 3/25xx	BP 118/78 120/70 Pulse 50 56
Prior Anesthesia 13 maxillary teeth extracted	Family Anes. Hx. Neg	Teeth up-good	Weight 240# 5-11
		Lower-front loose	

Allergies NONE   ETOH: Beer   Cig. 2PPD   Hepatitis Neg   Transfusions Neg

Medications   Neg

Phys Exam   Fx Maxilla R, Fx R Clavicle, T3-4 Fx unstable A2 no paralyzation, R AC dislocation, R Rib Fx

Anes Risk 2   SAB   Other risk explained to patient   some recall   NPO
             General   RA 7.4/33/62/24/1.9/89

Laboratory
Tx x 4   High GKPO4
EKG ? inf S waves   GRIP
Hct 42.6

Premedication   Effect   X RM Drake, MD   3/25/xx
   Neg   Anesthesiologist   Date

Pulse Ox				
O₂ Sat %	96			
ET CO₂ mmHg	31	32	30	33
Temp. C	34⁸	34³	34⁴	34³
EKG Lead	NSR	NSR	NSR	NSR
O₂ Analyzer %	90	91	91	90
Position	→	→	→	→
TIDAL Vol: cc	940	950	860	860
Rate/min	5	5	5	5
P.I.P. cm/H₂O	41	39	40	46
TIME:	5.	515	530	6.

IV Started
SAB Lot #   Exp:
MAC   O2   Nasal   Mask   INS
OPA   NPA   NET   OET
Miller   MAC   Stylet   LTA
ET Depth 22 cm   Secured IOR   Cuff
C Pressure   Pre-O₂   same

BG² 7.40/316/37/23/-1.8/9.6/11.1
5 – Pt autologous blood 1U given
6 – To Recovery
suctioned
extubation airway open
TORR
Awake
O₂ Sat 94
158/94
R18
P 90

Precordial

Esophageal

SCCA

J.R.

Bain

Eyes
Lube L R

Tape L R

PNS

Arms
Padded
L R

Anesthesia
Machine

6

6/0 5/180

Remark No:	BG²	5		6	X
O₂ L/M	2	2	2	2	
N2O L/M					
Foranel	1.1	0.5	2.5	0	0
Halothane					
Ethrane					
Pentothal					

Post OP Remarks

E.B.I.

Total Fluids:

RM Drake, MD   3.25.xx
Anesthesiologist Signature   Date/Time

RM Drake, MD C. Rodriguez   3/25/xx
Anesthesiologist/CRNA   Date

Anesthesia Record

Idaho Memorial Hospital

Idaho Memorial Hospital
876 Memory Lane, Anywhere, ID 83776
(208) 378-5555
Operating Room
Physical Assessment Data

Date: 3/25/xx

OR # 2

Operative Checklist

	Yes	No	NA
1. Identification Band Correct	√		
2. Lab Reports on Chart	√		
3. Surgical Consent Signed	√		
4. Consent in Agreement with Scheduled Procedure	√		
5. Allergies Noted on Chart	√		
6. Confirmation of Surgical Site and Side By patient response	√		

General Appearance

Pre Operative		Post Operative
____	Good Color - Skin Intact	√
____	Adequate Prep	√
√	Flushed	
____	Pale	√
____	Cyanotic	____
____	Jaundiced	____
____	Diaphoretic	____
____	Rash	____
____	Bruise	____
____	Reddened Area	____
____	Mottled	____

Observed Behavior

√ Cooperative	____ Restless
____ Crying	____ Resistive
____ Withdrawn	____ Combative
____ Talkative	____ Other

Post Operative Level of Consciousness

____ Alert	____ Non Responsive
____ Drowsy	____ Other
√ Responsive	

Cardiac Monitor ___yes___ O2 ___yes___

IV: See Anesthesia Records

Comments: Alert male to room via bed w/ neck brace on. RN at side during induction # 16 Foley into the bladder w/ clear yellow urine. Pressure boots to both legs. Positioned by Drs Manwise & Deery. Bovie pad site clear. Taken to recovery room w/o incident.

Signature: D. Johnson, RN   Date/Time: 3/25/xx 1820

Medications:

Drug	Dose	Method	Time	By Whom
See Anesthesia Record				

Time	O2 SAT	BP	PULSE	RESP
		/		
See Anesthesia Record		/		
		/		
		/		
		/		
		/		
		/		
		/		
		/		
		/		
		/		
		/		
		/		
		/		

Operating Room
Physical Assessment Data

Idaho Memorial Hospital
Anywhere, ID

<u>SURGICAL PRE-OPERATIVE CHECKLIST</u>

Patient's Age: __51__   Height: _____   Weight: __223.4__   Allergies: __NKA__

Has the patient ever experienced any previous problems with anesthesia?

Explain: __No_____

What routine medications does the patient currently take? __Colace - Peri-Colace_____

Does the patient have any pre-existing chronic condition of the heart, lungs? _____

Describe: _____

Has the patient ever had hepatitis: ____No____ When: _____

When did the patient last eat or drink?__2400_____3/24/xx_____

	YES	NO	N/A
Is the surgical permit signed?	X		
Has the prep been done?		X	
Is the ID band on the right wrist?	X		
Is the H & P on the chart or has it been dictated?	X		
Are the lab reports on the chart?	X		
Has the patient voided or is the catheter in place?	X		
Have the following been removed?			
Contact lenses	X		
False eyelashes			X
Wig, hairpiece			X
Eye prosthesis			X
Fingernail polish and makeup			X
All underclothing			X
Rings and other jewelry			X
Bobby pins, clips and hairnets			X
Dentures			X
Dental bridges and partial plates			X
Is the patient able to demonstrate effective coughing and deep breathing exercises?	X		
Is the patient able to demonstrate effective foot and leg exercises?	X		

Aprickboum, RN
_____

Signature of the nurse preparing the patient for OR

Young, Paul

Idaho Memorial Hospital
876 Memory Lane, Anywhere, ID 83776
(208) 378-5555

Physician's Orders & Progress Notes

Instructions: Notate progress of case, complications, change in diagnosis, condition on discharge, & instructions to patient.

Date & Time	Orders	X	Date & Time	Progress Notes
3/25/xx	May use Darvocet N1,00 in place of Darvocet N100 5.0			
Hold 3-25-xx MHawkins, RN	Dr. Manwise/H Caldwell LPN Patrick Manwise		3/26 0830	Stable VS- urine output ok Transport to ward
3/26/xx	Heparin lock flush 98 degrees Per critical care protocol. P. Elkins, RN Patrick Manwise			BX
3/26 0830	Ash Komylo to come adjust body Brace & fit chin/neck support pieces PT for ambulation walker, OOB as Tolerated in chair. Pneumatic boots While in bed Adv to reg diet, transfer to ward on Art linx. VS q4h Telemetry & nasal O_2 Cont all present orders Patrick Manwise Noted S. Dillon 0900			

x = only the prescribed medication may be dispensed.

Physician's Orders

Progress Notes

Idaho Memorial Hospital
876 Memory Lane, Anywhere, ID 83776
(208) 378-5555

Physician's Orders & Progress Notes

Instructions: Notate progress of case, complications, change in diagnosis, condition on discharge, & instructions to patient.

Date & Time	Orders	X	Date & Time	Progress Notes
3/25 1st dose 245 After in OR	Dr. Manwise's Postoperative orders: Vital signs c CMS checks post Recovery till stable the q4hours D51/2 NS c20 meq KCL/liter @125cc/hr heplock Respiratory Therapy to see IS QID ×5 days Physical Therapy to ambulate WALKER w/br out chin support for somi body jacket Lab: CBC qd ×1 day Nasal O$_2$ 3.5 l/min Medications: ANCEF 1 gm IVPB q6h Demerol 20-100 mg cPhenergan 15-25 gm IM q3-4 hr prn pain. Percodan i or ii po q3-4hr prn pain Darvon N 100 i or ii po q3hr prn pain Heparin 25 m u sq q6hr Dalmane 30 mg po qhs prn sleep Laxative of choice prn Colace 100 mg po x 30 days		3/25	Exploration & C7-T5 fusion & instrumentation Firdin fx pump locked facet - Impacted T2-T3 (L) - Bilat fort T3 Tx's - Fx port spinous Process & ® lower C7, T1, T2 Air wash to safely instrument zine For stability Patrick Manwise
Noted 3/25 @2000 MHawkins, RN	Call office to schedule return to office Appointment 2 weeks Resume all pre op meds Obtain Somi chin support From Reliah—Sicu tonite Log roll Sit to comfort Patrick Manwise			

x = only the prescribed medication may be dispensed.

Physician's Orders

Progress Notes

Idaho Memorial Hospital
876 Memory Lane, Anywhere, ID 83776
(208) 378-5555

Physician's Orders & Progress Notes

Instructions: Notate progress of case, complications, change in diagnosis, condition on discharge, & instructions to patient.

Date & Time	Orders	X	Date & Time	Progress Notes
3/26 1900	CBR SMAC)AM med Patrick Manwise 3/26/xx Noted Bwoods, RN 2030		3/26/xx 3-26-xx 30″ × 1 20″ × 2	Nutrition O: completed nutrition screening of medical record According to protocol.　　J Boresha, RD Physical Therapy – Pt is a 60YOM involved in a rollover about 2-3 weeks ago & suffered fx of thoracic spine. Also suffered AC separation ® shoulder Underwent exploration & ORIF & fusion of C7-T5 S: pt in much pain O: in AM, logrolled to ® side with max assist of 2 ® sidelying to sit with max of 2. PT sat about 5 minutes Then return to sidelying with max of 2 & logrolled with Max of 2. IN pm, logrolled & sat on edge of bed about 10 min while brace resituated down. Before supper Pt logrolled & to sit with max of 2. Sit to stand with mod assist of 2. Ambulated 5 steps forward and back with Walker & mod of 2. Returned to bed.
3/26	HCT 29 19 W Stable— Patrick Manwise			A: Tolerated fair. Pt reported that brace more comfortable When moved down. Chin piece in place for transfers. Some weakness in shoulders which was reported to Nursing, however pt states ® shoulder painful. Goals As stated & discussed with pt. STG 1 week 1. Pt perform logroll to sit to stand with assist of 1 2. Ambulate 25' w/ walker with assist of 1 3. Ambulate on stairs with mod assist of 1 P: will see pt TID for gt & transfer training. ------ K Whitcher, PT

x = only the prescribed medication may be dispensed.

Physician's Orders　　　　　　　　　　　　　　　　　　　　Progress Notes

Idaho Memorial Hospital
876 Memory Lane, Anywhere, ID 83776
(208) 378-5555

Physician's Orders & Progress Notes

Instructions: Notate progress of case, complications, change in diagnosis, condition on discharge, & instructions to patient.

Date & Time	Orders	X	Date & Time	Progress Notes
3/26/xx	Sr. V Bay or Dr. Lee to consult 3/27 ie pain in ® jaw		3/27/xx 20" gt	PT S: pt alert & cognitive O: OOB with logroll up to sitting with mod assist x2
3/26 Noted BWoods, RN	V.O. Dr. Man wise/ B. Woods, RN Patrick Manwise		Side rl off	standing with min assist 1. Amb. To hallway; back with Walker and cs assist of 2. Pt tol well tries easily. Up in chair for breakfast o nui—
3/27 Noted Paurlan, RN 100	Give ii units PRBC today T.O. Dr. Manwise/AU OR Paurlan, RN Patrick Manwise		3/27/xx	OS Consult Pt with hx of 3wk old trauma from AA- pt states Someone in T.F removed broken teeth & provided the Oral care. Exam now shows healing maxillary extraction Sites that are progressing satisfy. Pts CC is sore ® lateral
3/27/xx Noted Paurlan, RN 1400	1. Pt will need assistance w/tooth brushing of lower teeth Please do QID 2. warm saline rinses as tolerated by pt Qid Bret Lee			Border of tongue. Pt has flap of tongue which abrades over the teeth – there is a granulation bed on about 2 cm of lateral border – If there was not a recent trauma Hx, this would be highly suspicious for CA. Will Follow to wee if tissue tag will need trimming and Healing returns to normal appearance. Terrible oral
3/27/xx	De drain & change dressing May turn pt on side or stomach to DC drains of neck & back P.O. Dr. Manwise per SWITH Patrick Manwise			Hygiene present, but does not appear infected. Jaw intact -- Will follow pt____ Bret Lee

x = only the prescribed medication may be dispensed.

Physician's Orders   Progress Notes

Idaho Memorial Hospital
876 Memory Lane, Anywhere, ID 83776
(208) 378-5555

Physician's Orders & Progress Notes

Instructions: Notate progress of case, complications, change in diagnosis, condition on discharge, & instructions to patient.

Date & Time	Orders	X	Date & Time	Progress Notes
3/27/xx	Komy to Am to fit & mold now Custom body brace with Somi neck Extension. Make brace high in back & to manubum in front to immobilize		3/27/xx 20″ GTT +add ABD	PT –OOB with Mod (A) x2 via log roll. Sit to stand with Min (A) & amb with walker 50' CG. Pt in chair for supper with cast. ----- Trick, PT
	High thoracic spine Patrick Manwise		3/27	See oral surgeon notes. Afelnb-- Avon--
3/27/xx Noted BWoods, LPN	D/C O2 et tele d/c Foley @600am 3/28 V.O Dr. Manwise/ BWoods, LPN Patrick Manwise			Draining out. Patrick Manwise
			3/28	PT/ pt up in commode Amb in room with walker to door with Assist C/o discomfort with sitting in present brace. –klj;
			20″ gtt	PT/OOB with mod assist. Pt ambs about 60′ with RWR Pt c/o being shakey and hurting re: not to sit up for lunch Repositioned supine in bed & spoke with NSG, they Will transfer pt over to chair for lunch –Lwish, PTA

x = only the prescribed medication may be dispensed.

Physician's Orders   Progress Notes

Idaho Memorial Hospital
876 Memory Lane, Anywhere, ID 83776
(208) 378-5555

Physician's Orders & Progress Notes

Instructions: Notate progress of case, complications, change in diagnosis, condition on discharge, & instructions to patient.

Date & Time	Orders	X	Date & Time	Progress Notes
3/28 2030	CBC SMAC >call me w/results in AM Patrick Manwise One body jacket fitted on to shower Shell. Then back to bed, log roll To dry off & replace shell over T-shirt ------- Patrick Manwise Pm--Opsite one wound for grimes OT nerwerl 4 fx dry cheson Patrick Manwise		3/28 20″ gtt 3/28 2030	Pt-OOB with mod assist of 2. Pt amb with RWR about 60′ with Cg and returned to room. Pt put back to bed for brace adjustment ----- Trick, PT Stable no problems Has been fitted with body jacket would Heady fri pm Rv ok--- Stable and no apparent Problems Patrick Manwise
LFlower 2250				

x = only the prescribed medication may be dispensed.

Physician's Orders   Progress Notes

Idaho Memorial Hospital
876 Memory Lane, Anywhere, ID 83776
(208) 378-5555

Physician's Orders & Progress Notes

Instructions: Notate progress of case, complications, change in diagnosis, condition on discharge, & instructions to patient.

Date & Time	Orders	X	Date & Time	Progress Notes
3/28/xx Noted BWoods LPN 3/29/xx	D/C IV in am Velosef .5 gm po QID start am V.O. Dr. Manwise/ BWoods, LPN		3/29/xx 20″ gtt	PT/ pt OOB with mod (A) x1 & amb with RWR CG x 75′. Pt refused to sit up in chair due to shell 'digging' in his back. ----- Trick, PT
	Iron sulfate 0.3 gm p.o. tid T.O. Dr. Manwise/ L stami, RN Noted 12N Lstami, RN Patrick Manwise		3-29-92 20″ gtt	PT S: tired today. Says he sat up too much. O: transferred OOB with mod assist of 1. Amb 80' With rolling walker with CG assist. Sit to sidelying to supine with mod assist of 1. Po sitioned Onto side with assist of nursing A: Tolerated fair. P: Continues ------- KWhtiake, PT
			3-29-xx	P.T. –attempted to see pt for 3rd time; however pt had Been up for fitting of new brace & is tired out. Will See in AM. ------- Kwhtiake, PT
			3/30/xx	PT/pt brace was adjusted as ordered. Check chin brace & make sure in place. Before getting up for Dr. Manwise
			20″	Pt log roll OOB with min (A) & amb about 100' in hallway with walker & SBA & repositioned in bed Brace was loosened with assist from NSG. Tol well & feels better today. ---jenetBole, PT
			3/30/xx	PT/pt has been up with nsg in am due to nsg adjusting His brace. PT helped with transfer into bed & pt state. That he was too tired to Amb at this time. Will see again in pm. ---- JenetBole, PT

x = only the prescribed medication may be dispensed.

Physician's Orders   Progress Notes

Idaho Memorial Hospital
876 Memory Lane, Anywhere, ID 83776
(208) 378-5555

Physician's Orders & Progress Notes

Instructions: Notate progress of case, complications, change in diagnosis, condition on discharge, & instructions to patient.

Date & Time	Orders	X	Date & Time	Progress Notes
3/30 1720	Rehab consult plan transfer back to Rehab Mon if stable FeSo$_4$ 3 gm po tid Coumadin 15mg po today & Sun Do PT Mon AM & call w/results Patrick Manwise Noted BWoods, RN 2025		3/30/xx	PT/ pt OOB with min (A) & amb about 120' in hallway With SBA & repositioned in bed. Brace was adjusted as Ordered prn to amb. Tol well. will cont. --------janiceCole, RPT
			3/30 1720	138/3.7 94/11 HCT 28.8 Hgl 9.9— Stable Doing well Patrick Manwise
			3/31/xx 20″	PT/pt OOB with min (A) after brace was adjusted & amb 150' in hallway with SBA & positioned on Commode after amb. NSG later transferred to bed. Pt had A new brace put on last night to be C/O soreness and Being 'too tight'. Will cont to monitor soreness & adjust As necessary. JMATLOCK-RPT
			3/31/xx 20″	PT/pt's brace adjusted & OOB with min (A) & amb 150' w/SBA & positioned on commode. Toe better this Rx will cont ----- JMATLOCK-RPT

x = only the prescribed medication may be dispensed.

Physician's Orders   Progress Notes

Idaho Memorial Hospital
876 Memory Lane, Anywhere, ID 83776
(208) 378-5555

Physician's Orders & Progress Notes

Instructions: Notate progress of case, complications, change in diagnosis, condition on discharge, & instructions to patient.

Date & Time	Orders	X	Date & Time	Progress Notes
3/31 1230	Transfer to Rehab in AM----- Cont all present orders----- Call Kowry to adjust brace AM mon----- Patrick Manwise Noted 1435 labmi, RN		3/31 1230 3/31/xx	Trouble fitting brace comfortably -- Patrick Manwise PT/ S: Pt reports feeling 'good' today. O: Pt OOB with mod assist & brace adjusted properly. Amb with walker, CG I 85', Pt left sitting up on Commode. A: Pt tol TX well P: cont PT ----- jenetBole, PT ----- M Roholtz RTA
3/31/xx	Coumadin 5 mg po today d/c Heparin et ASA products T.O. Dr. Manwise Patrick Manwise noted Pdwilam, RN 1300		4/1/xx 20"	PT/ OOB with mod assist. Pt amb with walker about 80' with SBA. Returned to room requested to go back to bed Brace very bothersome. Redness noted Under ® armpit. NSG notified. ----- LWISH, PTA ---------- JenetBole, PT

x = only the prescribed medication may be dispensed.

Physician's Orders   Progress Notes

Idaho Memorial Hospital
876 Memory Lane, Anywhere, ID 83776
(208) 378-5555

Nursing Notes

Date	Time	Nursing Notes:
3/25/xx	1855	Received pt from RR via bed. Awake responding approp. Drowsy, dozes off to sleep Without stimuli. SOMI body jacket on. Chin support in room from rehab per Dr. Manwise request, outline patent (L) wrist covered with opsite. Clean dry no Edema. IV 051/2 NS patent @ 1ko in (L) arm with redness or edema. #7 from OR --#6 IV LR patent et inferring @ 125 degrees in ® arm tech vital without redness Or edema. HV ×2 draining dark red fluid #1 from neck + #2 (L) hip- graft site. Bilat ted hose on & bilat pneumatic boots on. Telem reading SR-ST c/o mild pain. Refuses pain med now. 20 c/o increased pain especially back of head where resting on brace. Felt used to pad brace. Demerol 50 mg with Phenergan 25 mg IM ® is for c/o pain.
	2045	decreased pain now sleeping quietly without distress before awakened
	2230	Requesting additional pain med explained ½ hour too early. Dr Man wise called
		About not being able to get chin support B/c have to tilt head back to far to get it on.
		Chin support off for the noc per md request.
	2300	Demerol 50 mg w/Phenergan 25 mg IM ® is for c/o (L) hip & neck pain. Lights off
		--- Hcaldese, lpn
	0000	Awake & c/o back pain. "Feels like I'm laying on needles." Alert & oriented x3. Moves all extremities well. Denies any numbness or loss of sensation. Radial, pedal & P tib pulses bilat equal & palpable 2-3+ with brisk capitia refill. Somi body jacket On. Dressing to neck, upper back & (L) hip & lower back in6tact. Hemovac to (L) hip and upper back intact. Opsite to (L) hip oozing small amt dk red blood. Lt radial Anterail line intact with good wave form. ® antecubital IV patent
		2300-0730 VELKNS, LPN

Nursing Notes

Idaho Memorial Hospital
876 Memory Lane, Anywhere, ID 83776
(208) 378-5555

Nursing Notes

Date	Time	Nursing Notes:
3/26/xx	11-7	Without edema or redness. LFA IV site patent with good blood return. Lt arm board
		On. Pneumatic boots on.
	0030	Log rolled to Rt & propped with pillows. Demerol 50 mg IM Rt thigh given for c/o
		Pain.
	0100	Neuro signs intact. States pain is now gone
	0200	Sleeping & talking in sleep off rom. Neuro signs unchanged. Has mild back pain.
	0300	Awake & requests change of position. Logrolled to Lt side. Side rails up ×2.
	0400	c/o mod. Pain mid back. Would rather roll further to Rt & helped to log roll &
		Propped with pillows. Assessment unchanged & neuro signs intact. Demerol
		75 mg & Phenergan 25 mg IM given. Lt thigh for c/o pain OU of LR empty & 14 g
		Angi cath left as heplock. Art line & LFA I intact.
	0500	Sleeping soundly.
	0530	Neuro signs intact. Dressings intact IV & at line intact.
	0615	Log rolled for sheets to be changed. To back
	0700	Sleeping off & on. VSS. Sinces rhythm without cctopy. Rate 90's neuro signs
		Remain intact. CMS intact ---- VElkins, RN

Nursing Notes

Idaho Memorial Hospital
876 Memory Lane, Anywhere, ID 83776
(208) 378-5555

Nursing Notes

Date	Time	Nursing Notes:
3/26/xx	0800	Awake, alert, temp ^100.1. Encouraged to deep breathe et cough et use IS.
		States slept 'ok' during night. Refused breakfast.
	0900	Percodan ii po give for c/o pain. States most pain in (L) hip graft site area.
		Hemovacs intact. Konmylor notified to come adjust SOMI brace.
	1015	To orthopeds per bed. Awake states pain pills helped his pain. On back at this time
		ART line dc'd. ® A.C. heplock dc'd. Heplock on (L) arm IV site ----- *Sidecer*

Nursing Notes

Idaho Memorial Hospital
876 Memory Lane, Anywhere, ID 83776
(208) 378-5555

Nursing Notes

Date		
3/26/xx	1945	Dr. Manwise notified pt c/o of pain in jaw by pt, Oral surgeon to consult tom — Bwoods, RN
	2400	V.S. taken –CMS checked unremarkable
	0130	Med with ii Percodan per pt request for inc pain- inc to DB—uses IS — Kjonson, LPN
		Relief with Percodan
	0200	Meds as ordered
	0500	Med with ii Percodan per pt request for inc pain – Relief --- Kjonson, LPN

Nursing Notes

Idaho Memorial Hospital
876 Memory Lane, Anywhere, ID 83776
(208) 378-5555

Nursing Notes

Date		
3/27/xx	0830	Up in chair for breakfast, ted hose on, chin brace on. Back to bed @0900, pneumatic
		Boots on, pt resting.
	1200	Lunch in bed. Didn't want to sit up in chair. Assisted with feeding, pt stated ® arm
		Hurt to feed himself.
	1300	Dr. Lee here for consult
	1345	2nd unit of pc's started, no reaction noted, pt sleeping.
	1430	Hemovac #1 & #2 dc'd. dressing changed. Blood infusion continuing without
		Problems. DJackson, SN ———— ---
		Neck incision clean & dry, drainage holes have sm amt of light red drainage, 4 × 4's,
		ABD & telfa in place with paper tape. (L) ihp incision clean with scant amt of red
		Drainage. Drain site hd sm amt of seous drainage. Pat tolerated entire procedure well 4 × 4's , ABD, & telfa in place with paper tape on (L) hip. Somi shell brace in place
		———— DJackson, SN ———— ---
	1600	PRBC transfusion complete without diff Nson
	1630	IVPB Ancef hang pt without s/s transfusion reaction denies c/o pain
	1645	Up in chair, requesting to go back to bed b/c too much pressure on back & neck when
		Sitting up that straight. Pt gt slow & steady with walker. Requires mod assist.
	1740	Percodan ii po for c/o neck & (L) hip pain given per RN. Tol 50% of meal fed per
		Nursing. Offer con't feed self b/c ® AC seperata cannot lift that arm
	1830	Sleeping quietly. HCaldwell, Lpn
	2000	Pt c/o mod severe pain in back/neck area. Medicated 2030 with ii Percodan per
		Request pain. Oral cares given. Pt's brace rubs into ® ribs. Padded with gauze
		Padding. HOB up 25% pt supine in proper alignment. States more comfortable 2/20
		O2/tele dc'd. 2200 pt. sleeping --- Scrane, RN
	2400	-0630 Slept on & off. Medicated for pain ×3. Turned ×2. c/o constipation-no BM
		Since before surgery -5 days. Dulcolax suppose. Given –stool felt in rectum. Foley
		Cath dc'd, urine dark amber. Encourage to drink. — RTuble

Nursing Notes

Idaho Memorial Hospital
876 Memory Lane, Anywhere, ID 83776
(208) 378-5555

Nursing Notes

Date		
3/30/xx	0800	Awake, up to ambulate with PT. Neck brace adjusted per orders.
	0915	Resting, states that body jacket is cutting him under arms et @ throat. Attempted to adjust jacket with mod relief of discomfort.
	1000	Otl bath given. Skin integrity beneath body jacket with reddened areas. (L) scapula et @ (L) waist. Jacket readjusted, drsg changed difficulty with positioning chin rest et
		Preventing jacket from pinching, incision line healing, clean et dry. Stockinette
		Changed beneath jacket
	1245	Up to commode, tol eating lunch while sitting up. Denies difficulty swallowing @ this time
	1430	Resting with eyes closed. Resp eupnic
	1430	Late entry. States has tingling on ® hand ,resolves with repositioning et movement at hand. --- A Levert
3/30	2400	Offer no c/o @ this time, voiding well. Amber in color. Needs assist with his urinal.
		States can't reach it has his new SOMI brace on. ----- L Fletcher

Nursing Notes

Idaho Memorial Hospital
876 Memory Lane, Anywhere, ID 83776
(208) 378-5555

Nursing Notes

Date		
3-29-xx	11-7	Slept well 0215 ii Percodan given with relief --- *CMenball, RN*

Nursing Notes

Idaho Memorial Hospital
876 Memory Lane, Anywhere, ID 83776
(208) 378-5555

Nursing Notes

Date		
3/31	2400	-0700 pt awake most of night watching tv. Requested pillow under his head.
4/1/xx		Placed a flat pillow under head. Appear to be resting better @ this time — Bmuir, Lpn

Nursing Notes

Idaho Memorial Hospital
876 Memory Lane, Anywhere, ID 83776
(208) 378-5555

Nursing Notes

Date		
4/1/xx		Repositioned for comfort. Denied need for pain medication.
	1530	Transferred to Rehab room 3915 via w/c. Personal belongings with pt. Report given
		By SN and LPN to charge nurse Rehab floor. Lungs clear, heart rhythm regular, no
		Edema noted. Back brace and chin plate in place. Cooperative and cheerful affect.
		---- MEliasen, LN -------
		RN tsf note: pt eager for transfer. Brace adjusted by Dea @ Komylo.no numbness/swelling reported. Cheerful affect. No problems noted Pdurlan, RN

Nursing Notes

Idaho Memorial Hospital
876 Memory Lane, Anywhere, ID 83776
(208) 378-5555

RESPIRATORY CARE OXYGEN RECORD

Diagnosis: Post OP

Date	Time	Modality	Lpm/FIO$_2$	On	Off	RT
03/25/xx	1900	NO$_2$	3.5	√	Bottle	S. Grasty, R.T
	2300	NO$_2$	3.5	√		M. Jacoby, RT
03/26/xx	0300	NO$_2$	3.5	√		M. Jacoby, RT
	0700	NO$_2$	3.5	√		V. Stewart, RT
	1100	NO$_2$	3.5	√		V. Stewart
	1800	NO$_2$	3.5	√		V. Stewart
	2300	NO$_2$	3.5	√		V. Stewart
03/27/xx	0300	NO$_2$	3.5	√		B. Davenport, RT
	0600	NO$_2$	3.5	√		B. Davenport, RT
	1100	NO$_2$	3.5	√		B. Davenport, RT
	1500	NO$_2$	3.5	√		B. Davenport, RT
03/28/xx	1020	NO$_2$	3.5	√		S. Grasty, R.T
DC'd						

Idaho Memorial Hospital
876 Memory Lane, Anywhere, ID 83776
(208) 378-5555

Respiratory Care Treatment Record

Diagnosis: Pre-OP/Post-OP T1-T12

Date __3/25/xx__ Time __0618__   Treatment Length __10__   Min   Medications __NS__
Incentive Spirometry _____   Pulse: Pre _____ Post _____   Couch: Productive _____   Non-Productive √
Ultrasonic Nebulizer _____   Sputum: Color _____ Approx Amount _____   Consistency _____
IPPB __Q4w/a__   Volumes _____ cc.   Peak Pressure __20cm/H_2O__
Small Volume Neb. _____   Breath Sounds __clear__
Chest P.T. _____   Comments: _____
Heated Aerosol _____   R.T __S. Grasty R.T__

Date __3/25/xx__ Time __1108__   Treatment Length __10__   Min   Medications __NSaline__
Incentive Spirometry _____   Pulse: Pre _____ Post _____   Couch: Productive _____   Non-Productive √
Ultrasonic Nebulizer _____   Sputum: Color _____ Approx Amount _____   Consistency _____
IPPB __Q4w/a__   Volumes _____ cc.   Peak Pressure _____
Small Volume Neb. _____   Breath Sounds __↓ R base otherwise clear__
Chest P.T. _____   Comments: _____
Heated Aerosol _____   R.T __M. Jacoby, RT__

Date __3/25/xx__ Time __2100__   Treatment Length __10__   Min   Medications __N-Saline__
Incentive Spirometry _____   Pulse: Pre _____ Post _____   Couch: Productive _____   Non-Productive √
Ultrasonic Nebulizer _____   Sputum: Color _____ Approx Amount _____   Consistency _____
IPPB _____   Volumes _____ cc.   Peak Pressure _____
Small Volume Neb. __Q2__   Breath Sounds _____
Chest P.T. _____   Comments: _____ **VOID**
Heated Aerosol _____   R.T √

Date __3/26/xx__ Time __0550__   Treatment Length __10__   Min   Medications _____
Incentive Spirometry __QID__   Pulse: Pre _____ Post _____   Couch: Productive _____   Non-Productive √
Ultrasonic Nebulizer _____   Sputum: Color _____ Approx Amount _____   Consistency _____
IPPB _____   Volumes __1000+__ cc.   Peak Pressure _____
Small Volume Neb. _____   Breath Sounds __clear__
Chest P.T. _____   Comments: __x20 Goals__
Heated Aerosol _____   R.T __V. Stewart, RT__

Date __3/26/xx__ Time __1100__   Treatment Length __10__   Min   Medications _____
Incentive Spirometry __QID__   Pulse: Pre _____ Post _____   Couch: Productive _____   Non-Productive √
Ultrasonic Nebulizer _____   Sputum: Color _____ Approx Amount _____   Consistency _____
IPPB _____   Volumes __1200__ cc.   Peak Pressure _____
Small Volume Neb. _____   Breath Sounds __Clear__
Chest P.T. _____   Comments: __x20 Goals__
Heated Aerosol _____   R.T __S. Grasty R.T__

Date __3/26/xx__ Time __1500__   Treatment Length __10__   Min   Medications _____
Incentive Spirometry __QID__   Pulse: Pre _____ Post _____   Couch: Productive _____   Non-Productive √
Ultrasonic Nebulizer _____   Sputum: Color _____ Approx Amount _____   Consistency _____
IPPB _____   Volumes _____ cc.   Peak Pressure _____
Small Volume Neb. _____   Breath Sounds __↓ R otherwise fairly clear__
Chest P.T. _____   Comments: __x20 Goals__
Heated Aerosol _____   R.T __M. Jacoby, RT__

Therapeutic Goals: Comments:
√   Prevent or treat Atelectasis
_____   Mobilization of secretions
_____   Deliver of aerosol medications
√   Improve ventilation

Idaho Memorial Hospital
876 Memory Lane, Anywhere, ID 83776
(208) 378-5555

Respiratory Care Treatment Record

Diagnosis: Post-OP T1-T12

Date __3/26/xx__ Time __1810__   Treatment Length __10__   Min   Medications __NS__
Incentive Spirometry __QID__   Pulse: Pre _____ Post _____   Couch: Productive _____   Non-Productive √
Ultrasonic Nebulizer _____   Sputum: Color _____   Approx Amount _____   Consistency _____
IPPB _____   Volumes __to 1250+__   cc.   Peak Pressure _____
Small Volume Neb. _____   Breath Sounds __clear__
Chest P.T. _____   Comments: __20 Goals__
Heated Aerosol _____   R.T   _S. Grasty R.T_

Date __3/27/xx__ Time __0625__   Treatment Length __10__   Min   Medications _____
Incentive Spirometry __QID__   Pulse: Pre _____ Post _____   Couch: Productive _____   Non-Productive √
Ultrasonic Nebulizer _____   Sputum: Color _____   Approx Amount _____   Consistency _____
IPPB _____   Volumes __1000__   cc.   Peak Pressure _____
Small Volume Neb. _____   Breath Sounds __pt in brace__
Chest P.T. _____   Comments: __20 Goals__
Heated Aerosol _____   R.T   _M. Jacoby, RT_

Date __3/27/xx__ Time __1100__   Treatment Length __10__   Min   Medications _____
Incentive Spirometry __QID__   Pulse: Pre _____ Post _____   Couch: Productive _____   Non-Productive √
Ultrasonic Nebulizer _____   Sputum: Color _____   Approx Amount _____   Consistency _____
IPPB _____   Volumes __1200__   cc.   Peak Pressure _____
Small Volume Neb. __Q2__   Breath Sounds __clear__
Chest P.T. _____   Comments: __20 Goals__
Heated Aerosol _____   R.T   _M. Jacoby, RT_

Date __3/27/xx__ Time __1500__   Treatment Length __10__   Min   Medications _____
Incentive Spirometry __QID__   Pulse: Pre _____ Post _____   Couch: Productive _____   Non-Productive _____
Ultrasonic Nebulizer _____   Sputum: Color _____   Approx Amount _____   Consistency _____
IPPB _____   Volumes __1200__   cc.   Peak Pressure _____
Small Volume Neb. _____   Breath Sounds __clear__
Chest P.T. _____   Comments: __x20 Goals__
Heated Aerosol _____   R.T   _V. Stewart, RT_

Date __3/27/xx__ Time __1900__   Treatment Length __10__   Min   Medications _____
Incentive Spirometry __QID__   Pulse: Pre _____ Post _____   Couch: Productive _____   Non-Productive _____
Ultrasonic Nebulizer _____   Sputum: Color _____   Approx Amount _____   Consistency _____
IPPB _____   Volumes __1000__   cc.   Peak Pressure _____
Small Volume Neb. _____   Breath Sounds __Clear__
Chest P.T. _____   Comments: __x20 Goals__
Heated Aerosol _____   R.T   _S. Grasty R.T_

Date __3/28/xx__ Time __0620__   Treatment Length __10__   Min   Medications __0__
Incentive Spirometry __QID__   Pulse: Pre _____ Post _____   Couch: Productive _____   Non-Productive √
Ultrasonic Nebulizer _____   Sputum: Color _____   Approx Amount _____   Consistency _____
IPPB _____   Volumes __to 1500__   cc.   Peak Pressure _____
Small Volume Neb. _____   Breath Sounds __clear to ↓__
Chest P.T. _____   Comments: __x20 Goals__
Heated Aerosol _____   R.T   _M. Jacoby, RT_

Therapeutic Goals: Comments:
√   Prevent or treat Atelectasis
_____   Mobilization of secretions
_____   Deliver of aerosol medications
√   Improve ventilation

Idaho Memorial Hospital
876 Memory Lane, Anywhere, ID 83776
(208) 378-5555

Respiratory Care Treatment Record

Diagnosis: Post-OP T1-T12

Date 3/28/xx Time 1020   Treatment Length 10   Min Medications 0
Incentive Spirometry QID   Pulse: Pre _____ Post _____ Couch: Productive _____ Non-Productive √
Ultrasonic Nebulizer _____   Sputum: Color _____ Approx Amount _____ Consistency _____
IPPB _____   Volumes to 1250+ _____ cc. Peak Pressure _____
Small Volume Neb. _____   Breath Sounds clear ↓ bases
Chest P.T. _____   Comments: 20 Goals
Heated Aerosol _____   R.T *S. Grasty R.T*

Date 3/28/xx Time 1500   Treatment Length 10   Min Medications _____
Incentive Spirometry QID   Pulse: Pre _____ Post _____ Couch: Productive _____ Non-Productive √
Ultrasonic Nebulizer _____   Sputum: Color _____ Approx Amount _____ Consistency _____
IPPB _____   Volumes 1500 + _____ cc. Peak Pressure _____
Small Volume Neb. _____   Breath Sounds clear to ↓
Chest P.T. _____   Comments: 20 Goals
Heated Aerosol _____   R.T *M. Jacoby, RT*

Date 3/28/xx Time 1920   Treatment Length 10   Min Medications _____
Incentive Spirometry QID   Pulse: Pre _____ Post _____ Couch: Productive _____ Non-Productive _____
Ultrasonic Nebulizer _____   Sputum: Color _____ Approx Amount _____ Consistency _____
IPPB _____   Volumes 1500 + _____ cc. Peak Pressure _____
Small Volume Neb. Q2   Breath Sounds clear bases
Chest P.T. _____   Comments: IS 20 Goals
Heated Aerosol _____   R.T *B. Davenport RT*

Date 3/29/xx Time 0635   Treatment Length 10   Min Medications _____
Incentive Spirometry QID   Pulse: Pre _____ Post _____ Couch: Productive _____ Non-Productive _____
Ultrasonic Nebulizer _____   Sputum: Color _____ Approx Amount _____ Consistency _____
IPPB _____   Volumes 1200 _____ cc. Peak Pressure _____
Small Volume Neb. _____   Breath Sounds clear
Chest P.T. _____   Comments: IS x20 Goals Self motivated w/ his own IS unit
Heated Aerosol _____   R.T *V. Stewart, RT*

Date 3/29/xx Time 1100   Treatment Length 10   Min Medications _____
Incentive Spirometry QID   Pulse: Pre _____ Post _____ Couch: Productive _____ Non-Productive _____
Ultrasonic Nebulizer _____   Sputum: Color _____ Approx Amount _____ Consistency _____
IPPB _____   Volumes 1500 _____ cc. Peak Pressure _____
Small Volume Neb. _____   Breath Sounds Clear
Chest P.T. _____   Comments: IS x20 Goals Pt doing IS on his own.
Heated Aerosol _____   R.T *S. Grasty R.T*

Date 3/29xx Time 1940   Treatment Length 10   Min Medications 0
Incentive Spirometry QID   Pulse: Pre _____ Post _____ Couch: Productive _____ Non-Productive _____
Ultrasonic Nebulizer _____   Sputum: Color _____ Approx Amount _____ Consistency _____
IPPB _____   Volumes to 1500 _____ cc. Peak Pressure _____
Small Volume Neb. _____   Breath Sounds clear to ↓
Chest P.T. _____   Comments: pt doing on own
Heated Aerosol _____   R.T *M. Jacoby, RT*

Therapeutic Goals: Comments:
√ _____ Prevent or treat Atelectasis
_____ Mobilization of secretions
_____ Deliver of aerosol medications
_____ Improve ventilation

Notes:

Notes:

Notes:

Notes:

Notes:

Notes:

Notes:

Notes:

Notes:

Notes:

Notes:

Notes:

Notes:

Notes: